Study Guide to Accompany
Radiobiology and Radiation Protection

Study Guide to Accompany
Radiobiology and Radiation Protection

Mosby's Radiographic Instructional Series

with illustrations

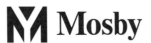

St. Louis Baltimore Boston Carlsbad Chicago Naples New York Philadelphia Portland
London Madrid Mexico City Singapore Sydney Tokyo Toronto Wiesbaden

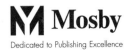

Executive Editor: Jeanne Rowland
Developmental Editor: Carole Glauser
Editorial Assistant: Jennifer Genett
Project Manager: Gayle May Morris

Copyright ©1999 by Mosby, Inc.

All rights reserved. No part of this publication may be reproduced, stored in a retrieval system, or transmitted in any form or by any means, electronic, mechanical, photocopying, recording, or otherwise, without prior permission from the publisher.

Printed in the United States of America
Editorial services provided by Wordbench
Scripting services provided by Tom Lochhaas
Composition by Wordbench

Mosby, Inc.
11830 Westline Industrial Drive
St. Louis, Missouri 63146

International Standard Book Number: 0-8151-5423-2

99 00 01 02 03 / 9 8 7 6 5 4 3 2 1

Reviewer

Mary Alice Statkiewicz-Sherer, A.S., R.T.(R), F.A.S.R.T.
Radiography Education and Medical Publishing Consultant
Imaging Professional
Summit Medical Center
Hermitage, Tennessee

Introduction

Radiobiology and Radiation Protection Study Guide is designed to accompany the Radiobiology and Radiation Protection multimedia program in *Mosby's Radiographic Instructional Series*. This study guide can be used with either the slide/audiotape or the CD-ROM version of the program. The multimedia portion of this instructional program, along with the study guide, will provide a solid foundation in the principles of radiobiology and radiation protection, radiation chemistry, cellular and systemic radiation effects, genetic and somatic effects, radiation detection and measurement, and patient and radiographer protection. The program can be used for both instruction and review.

The eight modules in this study guide correspond to the eight modules of the multimedia program. Usually you will find it more effective to experience the multimedia program first and then read and work through the accompanying module in the study guide. The different parts of each module in the study guide allow you to review and apply what you learn from the multimedia module as much or as little as you find helpful. Answers to the various exercises appear at the end of each module in the study guide.

Self-Assessment Pretest is a group of 10 multiple choice questions designed to help you determine how much of the module's material you have already mastered from the multimedia program before beginning to review this material in the study guide. If you incorrectly answered some questions, pay more attention to those subjects as you proceed through the other parts of the study guide.

Key Terms is a brief glossary section that defines important terms introduced in the multimedia module. It is important to gain a clear understanding of these terms and the concepts they represent before proceeding. Take a moment to read quickly through these definitions, and when you encounter items with which you are not yet comfortable, give special attention to their meaning. These terms will continue to be used in the following parts, helping you become more familiar with them and their importance in radiography.

Topical Outline presents in a brief format the primary information and knowledge covered by the multimedia module. As when reading the key terms definitions, pay particular attention to areas you are not confident you understand.

Review gives you a chance to interact with the material that has been briefly introduced through the Key Terms and Topical Outline sections. You are encouraged to write in the terms and phrases indicated by the blank lines in these descriptive and explanatory statements. Do not view this as a test. What is important in this exercise is that you are becoming more familiar with the terminology and concepts related to the module's content. Some artwork is included in this section, usually a variation of illustrations used in the multimedia program, to enhance the learning and retention of important concepts or processes.

Learning Quiz is unique among the various parts in that it is not intended to be used by those who have worked through the CD-ROM version of the multimedia program in what is called the interactive "student mode"—a student at the computer individually working through the learning program. In other words, you will want to complete this section if you viewed the slide-audio version or the CD-ROM program in "instructor" mode, without experiencing the program individually at the computer. If you have already worked through the full interactive program at the computer, you can, if you choose, skip over this section, which includes exercises you will have experienced already in the computer tutorial. On the other hand, repeating these exercises in the study guide format may be valuable as additional review. These exercises are designed to help you increase your mastery of the material by answering questions that require knowledge and understanding of key information that has been presented so far.

Applications addresses the module's concepts and information at a higher level by asking questions that require you to apply what you have learned in different situations or examples. This necessitates a fuller understanding of the material—how the principles of radiobiology and radiation protection apply to the specific topic. These questions are in some ways the most difficult in the module because they involve more than just defining terms or repeating information. Take your time with these. If you have difficulty, return to the Key Terms and Outline to review. If you do well in answering these questions, you probably have a good grasp of the material in this module.

Posttest is the final section in each module in the study guide. It consists of an average of 20 multiple choice questions designed to assess your understanding and retention of the information in the module after having worked through the preceding study guide sections. The answers to this section, unlike other sections, are not included in this study guide but are printed in the instructor's manual for the program—this is to allow your course instructor to use the posttest for more formal evaluation if desired.

This study guide is intended to make your learning experience more satisfying, while at the same time helping you learn, master, and remember what may be new or difficult material. The authors hope you find it an enjoyable experience.

Contents

1   Radiation Chemistry   1

2   Cellular Radiation Effects   23

3   Systemic Radiation Effects   49

4   Genetic Effects   73

5   Somatic Effects   95

6   Radiation Detection and Measurement   111

7   Patient Protection   131

8   Radiographer Protection   155

Study Guide to Accompany
Radiobiology and Radiation Protection

Radiation Chemistry

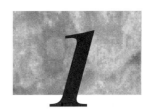

Self-Assessment Pretest

Before you begin to work through the Review, Learning Quiz, and Application exercises, use this pretest to assess your knowledge of the material in this module. Circle the best answer for each of the following questions. The answers are at the end of this module.

1. At what level does biologic damage resulting from ionizing radiation originate?
   a. Organic
   b. Cellular
   c. Molecular
   d. Organic and cellular

2. In what form is electromagnetic energy emitted from an x-ray tube?
   a. Photons
   b. Image-formation radiation
   c. Scatter
   d. Secondary radiation
   e. None of the above

3. What is the most important type of interaction between x-ray photons and body tissue?
   a. Compton scattering
   b. Pair absorption
   c. Coherent scattering
   d. Photoelectric absorption
   e. None of the above

4. What provides the contrast for proper imaging?
   a. Compton scattering
   b. All forms of scattering
   c. Photoelectric absorption
   d. Pair production

5. Which of the following statements is *incorrect*?
   a. The basic composition of the human body differs from that of nonliving matter.
   b. More than 85% of the human body is made up of hydrogen and oxygen.
   c. Carbon constitutes about 10% of the human body.
   d. Phosphorus and sulphur occur naturally in the human body.

6. What are the two states of water molecules in the human body?
   a. Anabolism and catabolism
   b. Free and disassociated
   c. Free and bound
   d. Metabolic and homeostatic

7. When does radiolysis of water occur?
   a. When Compton scattering occurs
   b. During metabolism
   c. During anabolism
   d. When water molecules are ionized

8. How long does it take for biologic damage to become apparent?
   a. Generally less than a week
   b. Hours to decades
   c. Within hours
   d. At least one generation

9. When is ionizing radiation harmful?
   a. During metabolism
   b. Within 10^{-15} seconds after a radiographic procedure
   c. When energy is transferred to atoms or molecules
   d. All of the above
   e. None of the above

10. What is the name of the standard measure for comparing different types of radiation and their biologic effects?
    a. Linear energy transfer (LET)
    b. Absorbed dose
    c. Electromagnetic radiation quantification
    d. Ionization density
    e. Relative biologic effectiveness (RBE)

Key Terms

Before continuing, be sure you can define the following key terms.

Absorbed dose: The measurement of radiation absorbed by an object, expressed in energy per unit mass.

Absorption: The transfer of x-ray energy to the atoms of the biologic matter through which it passes.

Anabolism: Constructive metabolism.

Atoms: Basic building blocks of all matter, including human tissue.

Catabolism: Destructive metabolism.

Coherent scattering: Scattering that results when a low-energy photon interacts with an atom and the atom responds by releasing the excess energy it has received in the form of a scattered photon.

Compton scattering: Scattering that results when an incoming x-ray photon interacts with a loosely bound outer-shell electron, dislodges it from its orbit, and then continues in a new direction.

Direct action: Occurs when ionized particles directly transfer energy to important macromolecules, resulting in the breaking of chemical bonds, which may cause biologic damage.

Fractionated dose: A dose delivered in equal fractions.

Free radical: An atom or molecule with a single electron in its outer shell.

Homeostasis: The maintenance of the body's internal temperature through perspiration and respiration.

Hydrogen peroxide: H_2O_2, a toxic substance that is poisonous to human cells.

Hydroperoxyl radical: A combination that can occur during radiolysis of water. Hydrogen free radicals interact with molecular oxygen, creating a hydroperoxyl radical. Hydrogen peroxide and the hydroperoxyl radical are considered the primary causes of biologic damage resulting from radiolysis of water.

Indirect action: Occurs when ionized particles interact initially with noncritical molecules, which are then broken down into smaller molecules, producing ions and free radicals that may recombine to form toxic substances, which can produce biologic damage.

Inorganic molecules: Compounds that do not contain carbon and occur in and outside the body.

K-edge: An abrupt increase in absorption that occurs when the x-ray energy equals the binding energy of the K-shell electrons in an atom.

Linear energy transfer (LET): The average energy deposited per unit length of the path or track of radiation; or the rate at which energy is transferred from ionizing radiation to soft tissue.

Macromolecules: Very large molecules consisting of hundreds of thousands of atoms.

Metabolism: Chemical and energy changes occurring in living matter.

Negatron: Negatively charged electron produced in a pair-production interaction.

Organic molecules: Life-supporting molecules; organic molecules contain some carbon.

Pair production: The production of a positron and negatron as a result of the interaction between a high-energy photon and the electrical field of the nucleus of an atom.

Photoelectric absorption: The result of the interaction between an x-ray photon and the inner-shell electron of an atom. The photon surrenders all its kinetic energy to the orbital electron and ceases to exist. The electron is then ejected from its inner shell, leaving a vacancy.

Photoelectron: The electron ejected from its inner shell atomic orbit (and thus absorbed) during the process of photoelectric absorption.

Point lesions: Injuries to molecules when chemical bonds are broken.

Positron: A positively charged electron.

Protracted dose: A dose delivered continuously at a low dose rate.

Radiolysis of water: The interaction of x-radiation with water.

Relative biologic effectiveness (RBE): The relative capability of radiations with different linear energy transfers (LETs) to produce a particular biologic reaction.

Scatter: The deflection of x-ray photons as they pass through the body after interacting with its atoms.

X-rays: Electromagnetic radiation emitted from the anode of an x-ray tube after bombardment of this target by high-speed electrons in a highly evacuated glass tube.

Topical Outline

The following material is covered in this module.

I. The interaction of x-radiation with the human body can result in biologic damage.
   A. Biologic damage occurs on three levels: molecular, cellular, and organic.
      1. The origins of cellular and organic damage begin at the molecular level.
      2. Atoms are the building blocks of all matter, including human tissue.
   B. X-ray exposure of patients can result in biologic damage to patients and/or imaging personnel.
   C. Absorption must be appropriate to produce a diagnostic radiograph without overexposing patients.
      1. Absorption results when x-ray energy is transferred to the atoms of biologic matter.
      2. Some absorption is desirable to produce contrasting images on the processed radiographic film.
   D. The basic radiation interactions include coherent scattering, pair production, photoelectric absorption, and Compton scattering.
      1. Coherent scattering is least likely to affect body tissue.
      2. Pair production does not occur at the energy levels used for diagnostic radiology.
      3. Photoelectric interaction, which is closely tied to biologic damage, is the most important type of interaction in the diagnostic energy range.
      4. Compton scattering, the second most important type of interaction, can endanger imaging personnel and can fog radiographic film.

II. The composition of the human body affects radiation absorption and biologic damage.
   A. The body is composed of five major types of molecules.
      1. Water comprises 80% to 85% of the body.
      2. The other four types of molecules—proteins, lipids, carbohydrates, and nucleic acids—consist of hundreds of thousands of atoms.
   B. Most molecules are inorganic compounds.
      1. Inorganic compounds do not include carbon.
      2. Inorganic compounds include water, acids, bases, and salts.
      3. Inorganic compounds occur naturally outside the body.
   C. Because of the abundance of water in the human body, it is likely to be a target of radiation interaction.
   D. Water plays a critical role inside and outside cells.
      1. Inside cells, water plays a crucial role in metabolism.
         a. Anabolism is constructive metabolism used to build up cell structures.
         b. Catabolism is destructive metabolism used to break down molecules.
      2. Outside cells, water supplies cells with external material and disposes of unneeded material.
III. Radiolysis of water occurs when water molecules in the human body are ionized by x-radiation.
   A. When ionized, water molecules dissociate into other molecular forms.
      1. Positively charged water molecules separate into a positively charged hydrogen ion and a hydroxyl radical.
      2. Negatively charged water molecules separate into a hydrogen radical and a negatively charged hydroxyl radical.
   B. After ionization, the free electron and ionized, positively charged water molecule may or may not recombine.
      1. If the free electron and ionized, positively charged water molecule recombine, no biologic damage occurs.
      2. If the free electron does not recombine with the ionized, charged water molecule, it can combine with other water molecules.
         a. If it joins another water molecule, a negatively charged water molecule results.
         b. The unstable, negatively charged water molecule can dissociate into smaller compounds.
   C. Both positively and negatively charged water molecules are unstable.
   D. Unstable atoms and molecules are more likely to chemically react with other molecules, causing biologic damage.
   E. Free radicals from organic molecules interact with oxygen to destroy molecules (causing biologic damage) and to form new free radicals.
   F. While an ionization event may take but a small fraction of a second, biologic damage can take hours to decades to become apparent.

IV. The degree of biologic damage is directly related to the amount of energy deposited along the track of radiation, a concept known as linear energy transfer (LET).
   A. Energy can be transferred to atoms or molecules, causing biologic damage, by direct or indirect action.
   B. Potential biologic damage increases as LET—a function of mass and charge—increases.
   C. Different types of radiation have different LETs.
   D. LET permits an assessment of potential biologic damage based on the number of ionizations that occur in a specific distance.
V. The relative biologic effectiveness (RBE) describes the relative capability of radiations with different linear energy transfer (LET) rates to produce biologic reactions.
   A. The x-ray, the standard measure of radiation, has an RBE of 1.
      1. Radiations with an RBE of less than 1 have a LET lower than that of diagnostic x-rays.
      2. Radiations with an RBE of more than 1 have a LET higher than that of diagnostic x-rays.
   B. RBE is expressed as the ratio of the dose of reference radiation quality necessary to produce the same biologic reaction in a given experiment.
   C. The longer it takes to administer a given dose, the lower the biologic effect.
      1. A dose delivered continuously at a low dose rate is called a protracted dose.
      2. A dose delivered in equal fractions is called a fractionated dose.

Review

Fill in the blank with the appropriate word or phrase. The answers are at the end of this module.

1. X-rays are _____ emitted from the anode of an x-ray tube after bombardment of this target by high-speed electrons in a highly evacuated glass tube.

2. When x-ray photons irradiate a patient, they may pass through the patient and produce a _____ image, they may interact with atoms or molecules of the body and be absorbed in _____, or they may _____.

3. Too little absorption results in a uniformly _____ radiographic image. Too much absorption results in a radiographic image without enough _____.

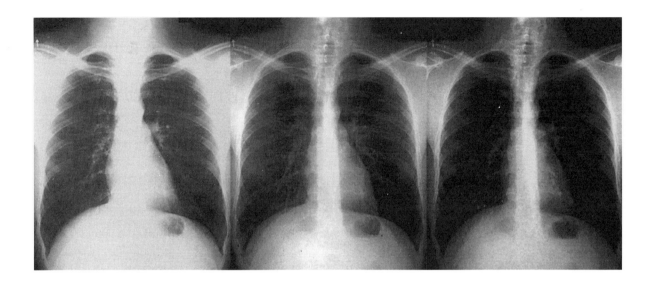

4. Too much absorption results in a higher radiation dose to the patient because patient exposure levels are related to the radiation that is _____, not the radiation that _____ the object being radiographed.

5. _____ x-ray photons are less easily absorbed than _____ x-ray photons.

6. The likelihood of absorption _____ as the average atomic number of tissue _____ and photon energy _____.

7. The biologic response to x-radiation usually depends on the four basic radiation interactions: _____ scattering, _____ scattering, _____ absorption, and _____ production.

8. The radiation interaction in the diagnostic imaging range least likely to affect body tissue is _____ scattering.

9. When an x-ray photon interacts with an inner-shell electron of an atom of biologic tissue, _____ absorption takes place.

10. An increase in photoelectric interactions signals an _____ in the absorbed dose of radiation. As the absorbed dose _____, the potential for a biologic response _____.

11. In x-ray images, bone appears _____, soft tissue appears as _____, and pockets of air (lungs and stomach) appear _____.

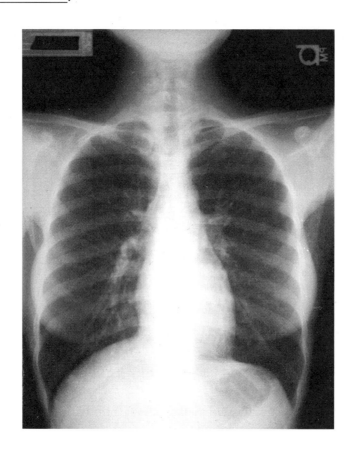

12. Photoelectric absorption depends on the _____ of the incident x-ray photons and the effective _____ of irradiated biologic matter.

13. Most of the scattered radiation during radiographic procedures results from _____.

14. Photoelectric interaction _____ as the energy of the incident photons _____.

15. The effective atomic number of biologic matter being irradiated affects the amount of radiation _____.

16. More than _____% of the human body is made up of hydrogen and oxygen.

17. Inorganic compounds include _____, _____, _____, and _____.

18. Salt compounds formed from the interaction of acids and bases are also known as _____.

19. Water consists of _____ of hydrogen and _____ of oxygen.

20. Water molecules that are independent of other molecules are in the _____ state. Water molecules attached to other molecules are in the _____ state.

21. Both positively and negatively charged water molecules are _____ and behave differently than unaffected _____ molecules.

22. When a free electron attaches to a water molecule, a _____ charged water molecule results.

23. A stable atom has an _____ number of electrons in the outer shell, also called _____ electrons.

24. The primary substances that produce biologic damage include hydrogen _____ and the _____ radical.

25. Excited atoms and molecules are temporarily _____ and likely to react chemically with other molecules, causing biologic damage.

26. Free radicals are formed from an unstable water _____ or from the interaction of the ejected _____ with another _____.

27. Molecules and ionizing radiation interact through either _____ or _____ action. Of the two, _____ action is the most common and may cause up to _____ % of biologic damage.

28. Biologic damage is primarily determined by the _____.

29. Linear energy transfer (LET) is a function of _____ and _____.

30. Equal absorbed doses of different types of radiation do not produce the same biologic effects because of the pattern of _____.

Learning Quiz

Some of the following learning questions are similar to the interactive exercises found in the CD-ROM version of this module operated in the "Student Mode." Please provide the best possible short answer. The answers are at the end of this module.

1. What are the risks and benefits of photoelectric interaction?

2. What makes a free radical unstable?

3. If a plant dies after irradiation by 6 gray of x-ray radiation and 4 gray of fast neutrons, what is the relative biologic effectiveness (RBE)?

Applications

The following questions ask you to apply the knowledge you have gained from this module. Please provide the best possible answer. The answers are at the end of this module.

1. Explain why there is a greater probability that compact bone (effective atomic number = 13.8) will absorb more radiation than an equal mass of soft tissue (effective atomic number = 7.4) in the radiographic kilovoltage range.

2. Describe the process of pair production. Why is this interaction generally *not* of great concern to radiographers?

3. What can happen when a Compton-scattered photon passes out of the patient's body?

4. What is the importance to radiologists of the abundance of water in the human body?

5. Describe the sequence of events in indirect action.

6. What is the scientific expression of linear energy transfer (LET)? What is the approximate LET of diagnostic x-rays?

7. What is the linear energy transfer (LET) of a photon emitted during a diagnostic x-ray? Explain why an electron set in motion by an x-ray has less potential for biologic damage than an alpha particle.

Posttest

Circle the best answer for each of the following questions. Your instructor has the correct answers.

1. What are the three levels of the biologic effect of radiation on humans?
    a. Genetic, molecular, cellular
    b. Organic, cellular, genetic
    c. Molecular, genetic, organic
    d. Molecular, cellular, organic

2. What is exit or image-formation radiation?
    a. Electrons that interact with atoms or molecules
    b. Photons absorbed in biologic tissue
    c. Photons that reach the radiographic image receptor
    d. Radioactive fog
    e. None of the above

3. What happens to photons that scatter as they pass through the body?
    a. They are deflected in a different direction.
    b. They continue through the body.
    c. They may reach the radiographic image receptor.
    d. They can be hazardous to imaging personnel.
    e. All of the above

4. What process occurs when the energy of an x-ray is transferred to the atoms of biologic matter?
    a. Biologic damage
    b. Uniform darkening of the radiographic image
    c. Uniform lightening of the radiographic image
    d. Absorption
    e. None of the above

5. In what parts of the body can radiation absorption take place?
    a. Skin
    b. Bone
    c. Tissue
    d. Organs
    e. All of the above

6. Radiation absorbed inside the patient is known as which of the following?
    a. Patient internal dose
    b. Soft tissue dose
    c. Absorbed dose
    d. Low-energy photon dose

14 Module 1: Radiation Chemistry

7. What occurs as the number of photoelectric interactions increases?
   a. The absorbed dose increases.
   b. The potential for a biologic response increases.
   c. The contrast of the radiographic image is improved at a lower kVp setting.
   d. All of the above
   e. None of the above

8. What is the general relationship between radiation absorption and x-ray energy?
   a. They are equal.
   b. Absorption increases as x-ray energy increases.
   c. Absorption decreases as x-ray energy increases.
   d. Absorption decreases as x-ray energy decreases.

9. What factors affect kVp selections?
   a. Type of examination
   b. Weight of patient
   c. Age of patient
   d. None of the above
   e. All of the above

10. What are the most abundant molecules or compounds in the body?
    a. Inorganic compounds
    b. Organic compounds
    c. Nucleic acids
    d. Lipids
    e. Macromolecules

11. What metabolic process takes place when the body needs to use the energy or substances it has stored?
    a. Catabolism
    b. Anabolism
    c. Homeostasis
    d. Scattering

12. What is the role of water in the body?
    a. Provides materials to cells
    b. Disposes of materials cells no longer need
    c. Dissolves acids, bases, and salts
    d. Helps keep bodies at a constant temperature
    e. All of the above

13. What happens when an x-ray interacts with and ionizes a molecule of water?
    a. Metabolism takes place.
    b. Anabolism takes place.
    c. An electron is dislodged, creating an ion pair.
    d. All of the above
    e. None of the above

14. What happens when a free electron combines with another water molecule?
    a. The free electron and the ionized water molecule recombine to form a stable, positively charged molecule.
    b. An unstable, negatively charged molecule results.
    c. The free electron and the ionized water molecule recombine to form an unstable, positively charged molecule.
    d. A stable, negatively charged molecule results.

15. What is missing from a positively charged molecule?
    a. A hydrogen ion
    b. A hydroxyl radical
    c. An electron
    d. An electron pair
    e. A hydroxyl ion and an electron pair

16. A negatively charged water molecule separates into what two components?
    a. Hydrogen ion and hydroxyl radical
    b. Hydrogen ion and hydroxyl ion
    c. Hydrogen radical and hydroxyl ion
    d. Hydrogen radical and hydroxyl radical

17. What are the hydrogen radical and hydroxyl radical also called?
    a. Hydroxyl ion and hydrogen ion
    b. Free electrons
    c. Free ions
    d. Free radicals

18. How do free radicals destroy chemical bonds?
    a. They transfer their excess energy to the molecules.
    b. They recombine to form a molecule of water.
    c. They form secondary hydroxyl and hydrogen radicals.
    d. All of the above
    e. None of the above

19. How do hydrogen and hydroxyl radicals cause biologic damage?
    a. They can destroy chemical bonds.
    b. Hydroxyl radicals can bond to form hydrogen peroxide.
    c. A hydrogen radical can interact with molecular oxygen, forming a hydroperoxyl radical.
    d. All of the above
    e. None of the above

20. What are the symbols for organic free radicals?
    a. R^* and H^*
    b. R^- and H^-
    c. R^+ and H^+
    d. RH^*

21. What happens when organic free radicals interact with oxygen?
    a. Biologic damage increases.
    b. Organic molecules are destroyed.
    c. RO_2 and HO_2 are formed.
    d. The free radicals interact with other organic molecules.
    e. All of the above

22. Free radicals can cause biologic damage by destroying the chemical bonds of molecules and by dislodging electrons from their orbits. How long will this process continue?
    a. Forever
    b. Until the energy reaches half of the initial energy
    c. Until the energy is lower than the energy of molecules they contact
    d. Until all the energy is expended

23. How long do free radicals exist?
    a. Hours
    b. Minutes
    c. 10^{-5} second
    d. 10^{+5} seconds

24. What results when macromolecules are ionized or excited by ionized particles?
    a. Chemical bonds are broken.
    b. Indirect action occurs.
    c. Metabolism occurs.
    d. Linear energy transfer (LET) occurs.

25. Why are most of the harmful effects of radiation the result of indirect action, rather than direct action?
    a. Most of the body is composed of vital molecules.
    b. Most of the body is composed of nonvital molecules.
    c. A free radical can damage only a single molecule.
    d. Biologic damage can take years to become apparent.

26. What affects the amount of biologic damage?
    a. Radiation dose received
    b. Type of tissue irradiated
    c. Amount of energy deposited along the radiation track
    d. Linear energy transfer (LET)
    e. All of the above

27. What increases the probability of biologic damage?
    a. Increased ionizations per micron of soft tissue
    b. Increased linear energy transfer (LET)
    c. Reduced speed of ionized particles
    d. Increased interaction between ionized particles and atoms and molecules
    e. All of the above

28. How do x-rays compare with alpha particles?
    a. X-rays are faster, with a greater mass.
    b. Alpha particles have greater mass, speed, and charge.
    c. X-rays are faster and produce fast electrons with a low charge and a small mass.
    d. X-rays produce more ionizations per micron.

29. Which of the following statements is *incorrect*?
    a. A dose of radiation delivered over a shorter period of time has a greater biologic effect than a dose delivered over a longer period of time.
    b. Linear energy transfer (LET) and relative biologic effectiveness (RBE) both affect the degree of radiation response.
    c. A dose delivered continuously is called a protracted dose.
    d. If the total doses of fractionated and protracted treatments are the same, the biologic effect is the same.

Answer Key

Answers to Pretest

1. c

2. a

3. d

4. c

5. a

6. c

7. d

8. b

9. c

10. e

Answers to Review

1. Electromagnetic radiation

2. Radiographic, biologic tissue, scatter

3. Dark, contrast

4. Absorbed, passes through

5. High-energy, low-energy

6. Increases, increases, decreases

7. Coherent, Compton, photoelectric, pair

8. Coherent

9. Photoelectric

10. Increase, increases, increases

11. White, shades of gray, black

12. Energy, atomic number

13. Compton scattering

14. Increases, decreases

15. Absorption

16. 85

17. Water, acids, bases, salts

18. Electrolytes

19. Two atoms, one atom

20. Disassociated, bound

21. Unstable, water

22. Negatively

23. Even, paired

24. Peroxide, hydroperoxyl

25. Unstable

26. Molecule, electron, molecule

27. Direct, indirect, indirect, 95

28. Radiation dose

29. Mass, charge

30. Energy distribution

Answers to Learning Quiz

1. Photoelectric interaction is closely tied to both biologic damage and image contrast. The absorbed dose—and thus the potential for biologic response—increases as the number of photoelectric interactions increase. On the other hand, photoelectric interaction helps produce contrast in radiographic images. Consequently, radiographers must weigh the risks and benefits of photoelectric interaction as they choose the energy level.

2. A free radical is unstable because of the missing electron in the outer shell. A stable atom has a pair of electrons in the outer shell, and the spin of one electron counteracts the spin of the other, balancing the atom. A free radical has just a single electron in the outer shell, and the single electron may spin in any direction, without any counterbalance.

3. The RBE is expressed as a ratio of the reference dose (conventionally, 250 kVp x-rays) to the other form of radiation (the fast neutrons, in this case): 6/4 or 1.5 RBE.

Answers to Applications

1. The probability of absorption increases as the average atomic number increases. The effective atomic number of compact bone (which contains calcium—atomic number 20—and phosphorous—atomic number 15) is greater than an equal mass of soft tissue (which is composed mostly of fats, containing large amounts of water).

2. In pair production, the energy of an incoming, high-energy photon is converted to two new particles—a positron and a negatron—as it nears the nucleus of an atom. Pair production occurs at energy levels higher than those used in diagnostic radiology, so it generally is of little concern to radiographers.

3. A Compton-scattered photon can interact with radiographic film—causing fogging—and it also can endanger radiographers or radiologists who are not protected. Protection of imaging personnel is as important as protection of patients.

4. Because water molecules are susceptible to radiation interaction and because there is an abundance of water in the human body (80% to 85%), the human body is likely to be a target of radiation interaction.

5. Indirect action begins when an x-ray photon strikes a nonvital molecule (such as a water molecule) and then proceeds to the creation of a free radical, to the interaction of the free radical with other molecules, to the destruction of chemical bonds on vital molecules, and finally to biologic damage.

6. LET is generally described in units of kiloelectron volts (keV) per micron of soft tissue, or keV/μm. The LET of diagnostic x-rays is about 3 keV/μm.

7. The LET equals zero unless the photon interacts with tissue and sets an electron in motion. X-rays produce fast electrons with a low charge and small mass, whereas alpha particles move more slowly and have greater mass and charge. Because of these differences, alpha particles can produce more ionizations per micron.

Cellular Radiation Effects

Self-Assessment Pretest

Before you begin to work through the Review, Learning Quiz, and Application exercises, use this pretest to assess your knowledge of the material in this module. Circle the best answer for each of the following questions. The answers are at the end of this module.

1. Which of the following statements about cells is *incorrect*?
   a. Cells occur in many sizes, shapes, and compositions.
   b. Cells control the growth and development of living matter.
   c. Cells compose the basic structure of living matter.
   d. Cells are the basic building blocks of all matter.
   e. Cells can act to protect themselves.

2. Name the four major structural components of a cell.
   a. Protein, cytoplasm, lipids, and nucleus
   b. Proteins, carbohydrates, lipids, and nucleic acid
   c. Cytoplasmic organelles, cytoplasm, nucleus, and membrane
   d. Membrane, nucleus, protoplasm, and protein

3. Where does DNA primarily exist?
   a. In protoplasm
   b. In the nucleus of a cell
   c. In ribonucleic acid
   d. In cytoplasm

4. What can occur after chromosome damage?
   a. Repair enzymes can reverse the damage.
   b. Cells, tissue, and organs can die.
   c. Abnormal metabolic activity can result.
   d. Cells can begin to multiply.
   e. All of the above

5. Where is energy for a cell produced?
   a. Mitochondria
   b. Nucleus
   c. Endoplasmic reticulum
   d. RNA

6. What are the two major components of a cell?
   a. Cytoplasm and cytoplasmic organelles
   b. Mitochondria and cytoplasm
   c. Nucleus and cytoplasm
   d. Centrosomes and the nucleus

7. What is the process by which somatic cells multiply?
   a. Interphase
   b. Mitosis
   c. Cell division
   d. Meiosis

8. How many chromosomes are contained in every healthy cell?
   a. 23
   b. 92
   c. 46
   d. 2

9. What is the target theory?
   a. An explanation for the interaction of DNA and RNA
   b. The differentiation between direct and indirect action
   c. The building-block theory of cell construction
   d. The presumption of a master molecule in each cell

10. What effect dose linear energy transfer (LET) have on the probability of radiation interacting with a molecule?
    a. The lower the LET, the greater the change of interaction.
    b. The higher the LET, the greater the chance of interaction.
    c. LET is not related to the probability of radiation interaction.
    d. LET affects only the probability of interaction in the presence of oxygen.

Key Terms

Before continuing, be sure you can define the following key terms.

Anaphase: The third phase of mitosis, when the duplicated centromeres travel along the mitotic spindle to opposite sides of the cell.

Apoptosis: A nonmitotic or nondivision form of cell death that occurs when cells die without attempting division during the interphase portion of the cell life cycle; also called *programmed cell death* or *interphase cell death*.

Carbohydrate: An organic compound responsible for providing the body with fuel for energy and serving as a structural component of cell walls and the material between cells. Carbohydrates consist entirely of carbon, oxygen, and hydrogen.

Cell membrane: The barrier between the cell interior and the outside environment that regulates the materials passing into and out of the cell.

Centrioles: The two hollow, cylindrical structures that result from the division of the centrome.

Centromere: The clear region on a chromosome that connects chromatids.

Centrosome: The central body of a cell, critical to cell reproduction; contains the centrioles.

Chromatid: A tightly coiled strand of DNA; also called *daughter chromosome*.

Chromosomes: Tiny, rod-shaped structures composed of genes.

Cytoplasm: The protoplasm that exists outside the nucleus of a cell.

Cytoplasmic organelles: Small components of cells contained in the cytoplasm that perform many functions of the cell.

Daughter chromosomes: The two sets of chromatids that develop during mitosis.

Deoxyribonucleic acid: DNA; the essential ingredient in chromosomes and carrier of the genetic code for cell reproduction and cell activity.

Direct action: Occurs when ionized particles directly transfer energy to important macromolecules, resulting in the breaking of chemical bonds, which may cause biologic damage.

Endoplasmic reticulum: Network of small tubes spread throughout a cell that serve as transportation routes.

Enzymatic protein: Protein that controls important chemical reactions within a cell by functioning as a catalyst; also known as enzymes.

G_1 phase: The phase of cell life cycle prior to the synthesis of DNA; the pre-synthesis phase.

G_2 phase: The phase of cell life cycle in which a cell prepares for mitosis by manufacturing protein and RNA molecules.

Gene: A segment of chromosomes; responsible for the formation of proteins.

Golgi apparatus: Tiny sacs located near the nucleus and tubes extending from the cell nucleus to the cell membrane; used both to make glycoproteins and to transport enzymes and hormones from the cell nucleus to the blood stream.

Indirect action: Occurs when ionized particles interact initially with noncritical molecules, which are then broken down into smaller molecules, producing both ions and free radicals that can recombine to form toxic substances, which can produce biologic damage.

Interphase: A collective term for pre-DNA synthesis, or G_1 phase; DNA synthesis, or S phase; and post-DNA synthesis, or G_2 phase.

Lysosome: Site where digestion occurs in a cell to eliminate waste.

Master molecule: The key DNA molecule in every cell, according to the "target theory."

Messenger RNA: RNA used by DNA to transmit genetic information; known as mRNA.

Meiosis: The process by which genetic cells or germ cells divide.

Metaphase: The second phase of mitosis, when the fibers of the mitotic spindle form between the centrioles.

Mitochondria: Site where macromolecules are digested by highly organized enzymes by the process of oxidation to produce energy for a cell.

Mitosis: The process by which somatic cells divide.

Mitotic death: Damage to a cell's ability to reproduce, which occurs after a cell has divided at least once; also called *genetic death*.

Mitotic delay: A temporary delay in mitosis caused by radiation exposure.

Mitotic spindles: The thin fibers that connect the centrioles on each side of the cell.

Oogenesis: Division of ova germ cells.

Ootid: The single functional daughter cell produced in the second meiotic division in oogenesis.

Prophase: The first phase of mitosis, during which DNA begins to take structural form and the nucleus membrane disappears.

Protein: An organic compound responsible for cell growth, cell repair, and new tissue formation; the most common organic compound found in the human body.

Protoplasm: The building material of cells that regulates the process of metabolism.

Ribonucleic acid: RNA; a type of nucleic acid used by DNA to transmit and arrange genetic information in the ribosomes.

Ribosomes: The site of protein synthesis in a cell.

S phase: The phase in cell division in which each DNA molecule is copied and replicated or divided into corresponding daughter DNA molecules.

Second polar bodies: The three nonfunctional cells produced in the second meiotic division in oogenesis.

Somatic cells: All the cells in the body except genetic cells.

Spermatogenesis: Division of sperm germ cells.

Structural protein: Protein that gives the body shape and form and produces heat and energy.

Target theory: The scientific theory that each cell contains a key, or master, molecule and that cell death occurs only if the master molecule is destroyed as a result of exposure to ionizing radiation.

Telophase: The last phase of mitosis, during which the chromatids uncoil and become long, loosely spiraled threads.

Transfer RNA molecule: Molecules that transport and arrange different amino acids according to the genetic code; known as tRNA.

Zygote: Fertilized ovum, produced when spermatozoa fertilizes the ootid.

Topical Outline

The following material is covered in this module.

I. Cells are the basic building blocks of living matter.
   A. Cells are made of protoplasm, which provides cells with oxygen and food and removes waste products.
   B. Protoplasm combines with other elements to produce organic and inorganic compounds.
   C. Cells control the growth of living matter.
   D. Cells are not equal.
      1. Cells vary widely in size, shape, and composition.
      2. Cells differ in their function.
      3. Cells reproduce at different rates, depending on type and age.
   E. Cells can remain stationary, move, reproduce, regenerate, grow, and defend themselves and other parts of the body.
   F. If cells are unable to function properly, the body cannot function properly.

II. The primary organic compounds are proteins, carbohydrates, lipids, and nucleic acids.
   A. Proteins account for up to 15% of cell material.
      1. The basic functions of proteins are cell growth, new tissue formation, and cell repair.
      2. Proteins differ from cell to cell, but the primary types are structural and enzymatic.
   B. Carbohydrates account for about 1% of the human cell.
      1. Carbohydrates provide the body fuel for energy, provide structure to cell walls, and serve as material between cells.
      2. Carbohydrates range from simple (monosaccharides) to complex (disaccharides and polysaccharides).
   C. Like carbohydrates, lipids (or fats) are composed of carbon, oxygen, and hydrogen; however, lipids have a much different structure.
      1. Lipids serve as stored energy for the body and protect the body and vital organs from trauma.
      2. Carbohydrates are a more efficient energy source than lipids.
   D. The macromolecules DNA and RNA are contained in the nucleic acids in cells.
      1. Deoxyribonucleic acid (DNA) is the source of the genetic code for cell reproduction and cell activity.
         a. DNA is the essential ingredient in the 46 human chromosomes.
         b. If chromosome damage is not reversed, cell—and possibly tissue and organ—death can result.
      2. Ribonucleic acid (RNA) is used to carry messenger (mRNA) and transfer (tRNA) DNA.

III. Cellular structure includes cell membrane, cytoplasm, and nucleus.
   A. Cell membrane protects the cell and controls the flow of material into and out of the cell.
   B. Cytoplasm, the protoplasm outside a cell nucleus, is the location of all metabolic activity of a cell. Cytoplasm contains a number of cytoplasmic organelles.
      1. The endoplasmic reticulum is a cell's transportation network.
      2. The Golgi apparatus both produces glycoproteins and transports enzymes and hormones.
      3. Energy for a cell is produced in the mitochondria.
      4. The lysosomes employ digestive enzymes to break down large molecules and eliminate waste from a cell.
      5. Amino acids transferred by RNA are synthesized into protein in the ribosome.
      6. The centrosome plays an important role in cell reproduction.
   C. The cell nucleus houses DNA and some RNA.
      1. The nucleus is the center of cell functioning, including cell division and bio chemical reactions.
      2. The nucleus is protected by two walls in the nuclear membrane.
IV. Different types of cells follow different types of cell division.
   A. Somatic cells divide by mitosis, whereas genetic or germ cells divide by meiosis.
   B. A somatic cell life cycle has four phases: pre-DNA synthesis, or G_1 phase; DNA synthesis, or S phase; post-DNA synthesis, or G_2 phase; and mitosis, or M phase.
      1. The G_1, S, and G_2 phases are also known as the interphase.
      2. The M phase has four subphases: prophase, metaphase, anaphase, and telophase.
      3. In mitosis, cell division concludes when two new cells are completed during the telophase.
   C. Genetic or germ cells are either male sperm cells or female ova cells.
      1. Cell division occurs through first and second meiotic division.
      2. A zygote results when two cells combine.
V. Many factors can influence the cellular effects of radiation, including the type of cell, where the cells struck, and the intensity and duration of irradiation.
   A. The impact of radiation on cells can be through direct or indirect action.
   B. According to the target theory, each cell contains a key or master molecule within the nucleus, a molecule presumed to be a DNA molecule.
      1. The location of the master molecule within the nucleus is uncertain.
      2. The master molecule has the same chance of being damaged as any other molecule.
      3. If the master molecule is destroyed by radiation, cell death will occur.
   C. Linear energy transfer (LET) and oxygen affect the likelihood of cell damage.
      1. The higher the LET, the shorter the distance between ionizations and the greater the chance of a molecule being struck by direct action. Higher LET also increases the probability that a molecule will be affected through indirect action.

2. The chance of interaction increases with low LET when oxygen is present.

D. Radiation damage can occur in a cell's DNA, cytoplasmic organelles, enzymes, and cellular fluids.

1. Damage to a cell's nucleus is the most serious cell damage, because the nucleus contains DNA. Damaged DNA can result in a loss of control over cell functions, can damage daughter cells, and can prevent cell reproduction.

2. Damage to parts of a cell other than DNA can interrupt or halt cell functions and can cause the production of toxic waste products that can poison or kill the cell.

E. Instant death of large numbers of cells can result from irradiation with a high 1000 gray (100,000 rad) dose of x-rays or gamma rays over a few seconds or minutes.

F. Reproductive death can result from exposure to a moderate dose of 1 to 10 gray (100 to 1000 rad) of ionizing radiation.

G. Cells react differently to radiation, with some more sensitive than others.

1. The intricate workings of cells are critical to the impact of radiation and resultant biologic damage.

2. The more a cell reproduces, the more radiosensitive it becomes (e.g., white blood cells, precursors of red blood cells, basal cells of the skin, intestinal crypt cells, developing nerve cells in an embryo-fetus, immature reproductive cells, and epithelial cells that line blood and lymphatic vessels).

3. Radioinsensitive cells include mature bone cells and cartilage, mature nerve cells, muscle cells, mature reproductive cells, mature red blood cells, and scar-tissue cells.

H. The 1906 Law of Bergonie and Tribondeau helps explain and predict cell radiosensitivity. This law states that the cells most sensitive to radiation are those that reproduce most quickly, have the longest mitotic cycle, are most immature, and have the least degree of specialization.

Review

Fill in the blank with the appropriate word or phrase. The answers are at the end of this module.

1. All functions of the human body result from functions of either _____ cells or _____ cells.

2. Radiation interferes with the proper _____ of cells.

3. The primary elements in protoplasm are _____, _____, _____, and _____. When combined with other elements, they produce the primary organic compounds: _____, _____, _____, and _____.

4. _____ and _____ are the most common inorganic compounds found in the body.

5. Cell characteristics are determined by the type of _____ in the cell.

6. Proteins are formed by combining _____ into long, chain-like molecular complexes.

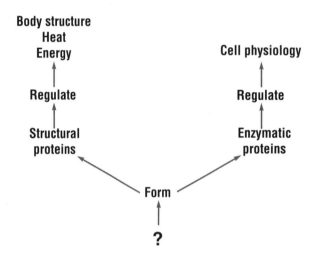

7. Carbohydrates, a vital source of _____ and _____, are composed of _____, _____, and _____.

8. Lipids are commonly found in great concentration _____.

9. The two nucleic acids contained in all cells are _____ acid (abbreviated _____) and _____ acid (abbreviated _____).

30   Module 2: Cellular Radiation Effects

10. DNA appears as two sugar phosphate chains in a _____ formation.

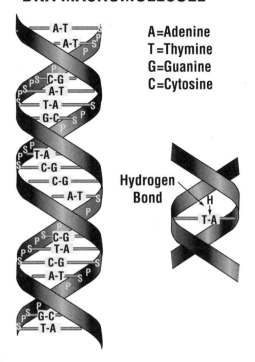

11. Segments of chromosomes, known as _____, are responsible for

    _____.

12. The cell _____ acts as a barrier between the cell _____

    and the _____ environment.

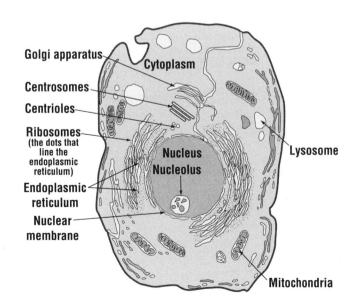

13. Cytoplasm exists _____ the nucleus of cells, whereas DNA exists _____ the nucleus of cells. The cytoplasm is the site of all the _____ functions of the cell.

14. The small components of cells suspended in cytoplasm are known as cytoplasmic _____.

15. All of a cell's cytoplasmic organelles are _____.

16. Digestion occurs in the mitochondria to produce _____ and in lysosomes to eliminate _____.

17. To produce protein, DNA in a cell's _____ sends amino acids to the _____ by messenger _____ (abbreviated _____) to be combined by transfer _____ (abbreviated _____).

18. The nucleus of a cell consists of _____, _____, and an RNA-filled _____.

19. Radiation _____ (does/does not) have to strike a vital point in a cell to cause biologic damage.

20. Cell division occurs through two phases: _____ for somatic cells and _____ for genetic cells or germ cells.

CELL LIFE CYCLE

21. During the _____ phase, a form of RNA is produced that is necessary for _____ synthesis.

22. DNA synthesis occurs during the _____ phase.

23. During the S phase, chromosomes change from two _____ connected to a _____ to four _____ connected to a _____.

24. Name the four subphases of mitosis: _____, _____, _____, _____.

25. During the _____ of mitosis, the _____ begins to take structural form.

26. During the _____ of mitosis, the nuclear membrane _____ and two _____ appear.

27. Germ cells are either male _____ cells or female _____ cells.

28. Direct action occurs when _____ interacts directly with _____, whereas indirect action occurs when _____ interacts with a _____. Damage is most severe when the nucleus is damaged, because it contains _____.

DIRECT ACTION

INDIRECT ACTION

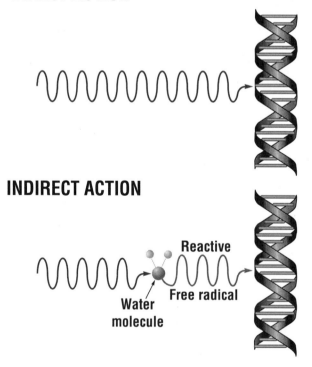

34 Module 2: Cellular Radiation Effects

29. According to target theory, cell death due to destruction of the master molecule can occur by either _____ or _____ action.

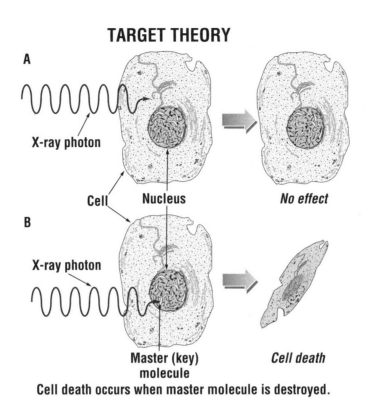

TARGET THEORY

Cell death occurs when master molecule is destroyed.

30. With low linear energy transfer (LET), the probability of radiation interaction increases when _____ is present because of the formation of reactive free _____. When damage occurs through an oxygenated process, the damage is _____.

31. Cell damage repair is most likely with _____ linear energy transfer (LET) and low _____ rates.

Module 2: Cellular Radiation Effects 35

Learning Quiz

Some of the following learning questions are similar to the interactive exercises found in the CD-ROM version of this module operated in the "Student Mode." Please provide the best possible short answer. The answers are at the end of this module.

1. Explain how genetic code is transmitted from DNA via messenger RNA (mRNA) to transfer RNA (tRNA). What happens if DNA, mRNA, or tRNA are interrupted?

2. Why is the role of lysosomes important to radiographic imaging?

3. Describe the basic phases in the cell life cycle, including interphase and cell division.

Applications

The following questions ask you to apply the knowledge you have gained from this module. Please provide the best possible answer. The answers are at the end of this module.

1. Explain why lipids are a greater problem in regulating body weight than carbohydrates.

2. How does DNA regulate the way each of us looks—that is, our body size, shape, and features?

3. What is the role of DNA in radiation-induced malignant disease?

4. Why is radiation damage to the cell nucleus so serious? Why is the interaction of radiation with water molecules within a cell so important in radiographic imaging?

5. How does germ cell division differ from somatic cell division?

6. Explain the target theory. How is it affected by direct and indirect action?

7. What doses of radiation cause instant death? Reproductive death? How do these differ from mitotic delay?

8. Explain the Law of Bergonie and Tribondeau. Give examples of highly sensitive and highly insensitive cells.

Posttest

Circle the best answer for each of the following questions. Your instructor has the correct answers.

1. Which of the following statements best describes cells?
   a. Cells occur in many sizes, shapes, and compositions.
   b. Cell are microscopic and uniform in size and shape.
   c. Cells vary in size and shape but have uniform composition.
   d. Cells are microscopic and uniform in composition.

2. What can result when radiation interferes with cell function by damaging the cell's nucleus?
   a. Chromosome breakage
   b. Instant cell death
   c. Reproductive death
   d. Interference of function
   e. All of the above

3. What are cells composed of?
   a. Oxygen, nitrogen, and carbon only
   b. Protoplasm
   c. Lipids only
   d. Carbohydrates only

4. What is the most common organic compound in the human body?
   a. Lipid
   b. Carbohydrate
   c. Protein
   d. Nucleic acid

5. What are the functions of proteins?
   a. Serving as hormones and antibodies
   b. Building tissue and regulating body development
   c. Regulating body development and protecting against illness
   d. Promoting cell growth and repairing damaged and debilitated cells
   e. All of the above

6. What is a key role of carbohydrates?
   a. Facilitating cell growth
   b. Protecting vital organs from trauma
   c. Regulating the body's shape
   d. Providing the body fuel for energy

7. Which of the following statements about carbohydrates and lipids is *incorrect*?
   a. Both are composed of carbon, oxygen, and hydrogen.
   b. Both serve as an energy source for the body.
   c. Both protect the body from temperature extremes.
   d. Both are a structural component of cells.
   e. All of the above

8. What is the function of cell membrane?
   a. Regulating the flow of material into a cell
   b. Regulating the flow of material out of a cell
   c. Determining what material should be permitted into or out of a cell
   d. All of the above
   e. None of the above

9. What occurs in the passive mode of transportation through the cell membrane?
   a. Material does not flow into the cell.
   b. Material does not flow out of the cell.
   c. Material moves through the membrane by osmosis.
   d. Answers (a) and (b) only
   e. None of the above

10. What is the primary material inside a cell?
    a. Cytoplasm
    b. RNA
    c. Passive membrane
    d. DNA

11. What is the term for the network of tubes in a cell that transports food, waste products, and mRNA?
    a. Protoplasm
    b. Cytoplasm
    c. Golgi apparatus
    d. Endoplasmic reticulum

12. Approximately what percentage of the body consists of proteins?
    a. 0.75%
    b. 3.5%
    c. 15%
    d. 35%

13. Which cytoplasmic organelle affects the formation of the mitotic spindle?
    a. Centrosome
    b. Endoplasmic reticulum
    c. Golgi apparatus
    d. Mitochondria

14. Which part of a cell contains DNA?
    a. Cytoplasm
    b. Centrosome
    c. Messenger RNA
    d. Nucleus
    e. Endoplasmic reticulum

15. What is the DNA messenger?
    a. tRNA
    b. mRNA
    c. Ribosome
    d. Centrome
    e. All of the above

16. Why does the cell nucleus have two walls?
    a. To protect the nucleus and connect the nucleolus and the endoplasmic reticulum tubes
    b. To store RNA
    c. To house DNA
    d. To direct the synthesis of protein
    e. All of the above

17. What occurs when a cytoplasmic organelle is damaged?
    a. Cell death
    b. Permanent cell damage
    c. Damage to all other cytoplasmic organelles
    d. Cell death or cell repair and recovery

18. What is another term for the G_1 phase?
    a. Interphase
    b. Prophase
    c. Pre-DNA synthesis phase
    d. Mitosis

19. What structures having identical DNA are formed during the S phase?
    a. Two pairs of chromatids
    b. Two pairs of centromeres
    c. Two chromosomes
    d. Two strands of DNA

20. What occurs during the G_2 phase?
    a. The cell prepares for mitosis.
    b. The cell manufactures protein.
    c. RNA molecules are produced.
    d. All of the above
    e. None of the above

21. What are centrioles?
    a. Centrosomes
    b. Centrosomes that have divided into two parts
    c. Divided mitotic spindles
    d. Chromatids that have multiplied
    e. None of the above

22. What is the function of the centrioles?
    a. Producing protein
    b. Protecting the nucleus
    c. Regulating the formation of mitotic spindle
    d. Forming a connection to the centromere

23. What occurs during metaphase, the second phase of mitosis?
    a. The centrome divides into two centrioles.
    b. The cell nucleus separates.
    c. The centromeres are duplicated.
    d. All of the above
    e. None of the above

24. The four chromatids that developed during the S phase split into a two-chromatid structure during what phase?
    a. Anaphase
    b. Metaphase
    c. Interphase
    d. Prophase

25. In what phase of mitosis do chromatids (or daughter chromosomes) uncoil and become fully functional chromosomes?
    a. Anaphase
    b. Prophase
    c. Metaphase
    d. Telophase

26. Where is the master molecule located?
    a. Generally in the cytoplasm
    b. Always in the nucleus
    c. Anywhere within the cell
    d. Always in the cytoplasm

27. What are the effects of radiation damage to DNA?
    a. Loss of control over cell function
    b. Daughter cells with greater loss of cell function
    c. Compromised ability to divide or reproduce
    d. Any of the above
    e. None of the above

28. When does most cell damage occur?
    a. When a master molecule interacts directly with radiation
    b. When a master molecule interacts indirectly with radiation
    c. When a molecule other than a master molecule interacts with radiation
    d. Answers (a) and (b) only
    e. None of the above

29. What is generally the most serious type of cell damage?
    a. Chromosome breakage
    b. Cell function damage
    c. Cell function interference
    d. Mitotic delay

30. Which of the following statements is *incorrect*?
    a. Different cells react differently to radiation.
    b. Some cells repair damage better than others.
    c. Some cells replace damaged cells better than others.
    d. The radiosensitivity of cells is equal.
    e. Different organs are more susceptible to radiation damage than others.

Answer Key

Answers to Pretest

1. d
2. c
3. b
4. e
5. a
6. c
7. b
8. c
9. d
10. b

Answers to Review

1. Individual, groups of
2. Functioning
3. Oxygen, nitrogen, carbon, hydrogen, proteins, carbohydrates, lipids, nucleic acids
4. Water, mineral salts
5. Protein
6. Amino acids
7. Starches, sugars, carbon, oxygen, hydrogen
8. Just beneath the skin
9. Deoxyribonucleic, DNA, ribonucleic, RNA
10. Twisted helix
11. Genes, heredity
12. Membrane, interior, outside
13. Outside, inside, metabolic
14. Organelles
15. Interrelated
16. Energy, waste
17. Nucleus, ribosome, RNA, mRNA, RNA, tRNA
18. Protoplasm, DNA, nucleolus
19. Does not
20. Mitosis, meiosis
21. G_1, DNA
22. S
23. Chromatids, centromere, chromatids, centromere

24. Prophase, metaphase, anaphase, telophase

25. Prophase, DNA

26. Telophase, reforms, nuclei

27. Sperm, ova

28. Radiation, vital macromolecules, radiation, noncritical molecule, DNA

29. Direct, indirect

30. Oxygen, radicals, permanent

31. Low, dose

Answers to Learning Quiz

1. mRNA carries genetic codes from DNA (which is located in the nucleus of a cell) through a network of canals to ribosomes, where proteins are produced. mRNA then gives the genetic code to 1 of 22 tRNA molecules, which transport and arrange amino acids according to the code. Interruption of this process affects the production of protein, which can threaten the survival of the cell.

2. The digestive enzymes in the lysosomes are toxic to cells. Radiation can cause a lysosome sac to rupture, which will poison and kill the cell.

3. Somatic cells divide by mitosis, whereas genetic or germ cells divide by meiosis. The interphase—the pre-DNA synthesis, or G_1 phase; DNA synthesis, or S phase; and post-DNA synthesis, or G_2 phase—occurs before the mitosis or M phase. The M phase has four subphases: prophase, metaphase, anaphase, and telophase.

Answers to Applications

1. Although lipids and carbohydrates are composed of the same three elements—carbon, oxygen, and hydrogen—their structure and their functions are quite different. Lipids are not converted to energy as easily as are carbohydrates; thus the body uses carbohydrates for energy before lipids during exercise.

2. DNA regulates the sequences of amino acids in proteins. Because proteins provide structure and support for the body, and because DNA directs where that support and structure should go, DNA regulates body shape, size, and characteristics.

3. DNA damage can result in abnormal metabolic activity, resulting in cell growth.

4. The most serious damage to a cell occurs when the nucleus is affected, because it can interfere with protein production as well as DNA message transfer via mRNA and can even cause chromosome damage. Since most of a cell consists of water, the chances are high that an x-ray photon will strike a water molecule, which can set off a chain reaction of interactions resulting in cell damage or cell death.

5. Division is similar to the point that the two daughter cells are produced. At this point, the daughter cells divide again; however in germ cells the daughter cells split the DNA rather than duplicating it. The result is four daughter cells in germ cells, each with 23 chromosomes. These daughter cells then unite with sperm or ova, each of which also contains 23 chromosomes, to produce a zygote, or fertilized ovum.

6. Target theory—which has not been proven—postulates that each cell contains a master, or key, molecule. For cell death to occur, this master molecule must be destroyed. The master molecule does not have to be hit directly; it can be destroyed through indirect action.

7. Instant death of large numbers of cells can result from irradiation with a high 1000 gray (100,000 rad) dose of x-rays or gamma rays over a period of a few seconds to a few minutes. (This dose is much higher than the range used in diagnostic and therapeutic treatment.) Reproductive death can result from irradiation with a moderate 1 to 10 gray (100 to 1000 rad) dose of ionizing radiation. In mitotic delay, mitosis is delayed in a cell exposed to radiation just before dividing; if the cell is otherwise undamaged, division will resume normally.

8. The 1906 Law of Bergonie and Tribondeau states that radiosensitivity is directly proportional to a cell's reproductive activity and inversely proportional to a cell's degree of differentiation. Cells that reproduce most quickly, have the longest mitotic cycle, are most immature, and have the lowest degree of specification are most sensitive to radiation, whereas cells that reproduce slowly, have the shortest mitotic cycles, are mature, and have a high degree of specification are least sensitive to radiation. Cells with a high sensitivity include white blood cells, precursors of red blood cells, basal cells of the skin, intestinal crypt cells, developing nerve cells in an embryo or fetus, immature reproductive cells, and epithelial cells that line blood and lymphatic vessels. Cells with a low sensitivity include mature bone cells and cartilage, mature nerve cells, muscle cells, mature reproductive cells, mature red blood cells, and scar tissue cells.

Systemic Radiation Effects

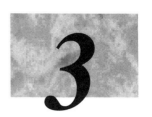

Self-Assessment Pretest

Before you begin to work through the Review, Learning Quiz, and Application exercises, use this pretest to assess your knowledge of the material in this module. Circle the best answer for each of the following questions. The answers are at the end of this module.

1. When do the early somatic effects of a substantial dose of radiation occur?
    a. Within seconds of exposure
    b. Months to years after exposure
    c. From minutes to weeks after exposure
    d. After 1 or 2 generations

2. What does a linear nonthreshold radiation dose-response relationship indicate?
    a. The relationship between radiation dose and biologic response is directly proportional.
    b. No threshold exists at which radiation causes any biologic effect.
    c. The biologic response is the same, regardless of the radiation dose.
    d. The same radiation dose can give a range of biologic responses.

3. What happens in the final stage of acute radiation syndrome?
    a. Death always
    b. Recovery always
    c. Chronic illness
    d. Either death or recovery
    e. None of the above

4. What dose defines the beginning of the acute radiation syndrome?
    a. 10 Gy (1000 rad)
    b. 1 Gy (100 rad)
    c. 100 Gy (10,000 rad)
    d. 0.1 Gy (10 rad)

5. What is the most radiosensitive organ or system in the human body?
    a. Thymus
    b. Spleen
    c. Erythrocytes
    d. Hematopoietic
    e. Leukocytes

6. Where are most blood cells manufactured?
   a. Thymus
   b. Gastrointestinal system
   c. Bone marrow
   d. Cardiovascular system

7. What are the most numerous of all blood cells?
   a. Erythrocytes
   b. Leukocytes
   c. Stem cells
   d. Platelet cells

8. What is the expected survival time for individuals exposed to whole-body radiation of more than 6 Gy (600 rad)?
   a. Normal life expectancy with proper treatment
   b. Months to years
   c. Weeks to months
   d. Normally less than 2 weeks

9. Above what dose of ionizing radiation does the cerebrovascular syndrome begin to occur?
   a. 500 Gy (50,000 rad)
   b. 50 Gy (5000 rad)
   c. 5 Gy (500 rad)
   d. 15 Gy (1500 rad)

10. What happens to the radiosensitivity of an embryo-fetus as it ages?
    a. Stays the same
    b. Increases exponentially
    c. Increases steadily
    d. Decreases

Key Terms

Before continuing, be sure you can define the following key terms.

Acute radiation syndrome (ARS): The result of whole-body exposure to large doses of ionizing radiation (1Gy [100 rad] or more) over a short period; symptoms include nausea, blood disorders, intestinal disorders, fever, fatigue, sperm count depression, temporary or permanent sterility in both sexes, cardiovascular system damage, central nervous system damage, and skin shedding.

Cerebrovascular syndrome: A form of acute radiation syndrome that occurs when an individual receives a whole-body absorbed dose of ionizing radiation above 50 Gy (5000 rad); also known as *central nervous system syndrome*.

Dose-response relationship: Relationship between levels of radiation doses and the degree of observed biologic response.

Electrolytes: Solutions capable of conducting electricity.

Erythrocytes: A type of red blood cell and the most numerous of all blood cells.

Gastrointestinal syndrome: A form of acute radiation syndrome that occurs in humans when an individual receives a whole-body threshold dose of ionizing radiation of approximately 6 Gy (600 rad).

Hematopoietic syndrome: A form of acute radiation syndrome that occurs when an individual receives a whole-body dose of ionizing radiation of 1 to 10 Gy (100 to 1000 rad); also known as *bone-marrow syndrome*.

LD 50/30: The whole-body radiation dose at which 50% of the individuals exposed will die within 30 days.

Linear energy transfer (LET): Average energy deposited per unit length of the path or track of radiation or the rate at which energy is transferred from ionizing radiation to soft tissue.

Linear response: A response which is directly proportional to radiation dose; as dose increases, the response rises in equally measured increments.

Lymphocytes: A type of white blood cell and the most radiosensistive of all blood cells in the human body; lymphocytes help protect the body from disease.

Mean survival time: The average survival time between radiation exposure and death.

Nonlinear response: A response that is not directly proportional to radiation dose.

Nonthreshold: The assumption that a response to radiation exposure will occur at any dose, as in a nonthreshold dose-response relationship.

Platelets: Blood cells that allow blood clotting and stop hemorrhage; also called *thrombocytes*.

Syndrome: Medical term for a collection of symptoms, such as acute radiation syndrome.

Threshold: A point at which a biologic response to radiation first occurs, as in a threshold radiation dose-response relationship.

Villi: Columns of cells lining the intestinal lining.

Topical Outline

The following material is covered in this module.

I. The radiation dose-response relationship is the relationship between radiation exposure and observed response.
   A. Understanding the radiation dose-response relationship is necessary for using radiation as therapy for malignant diseases.
   B. Understanding the radiation dose-response relationship is necessary to understand the effects of low-dose radiation.
   C. Dose-response relationships have two characteristics.
      1. Dose-response relationships are either linear (straight line) or nonlinear (curved line).
      2. Dose-response relationships are either threshold (indicating a point at which a response to radiation first occurs) or nonthreshold (indicating that a response could occur at any dose).
   D. The linear-quadratic nonthreshold curve on a graph of dose-response relationships indicates that as dose increases at a given rate, the response increases more rapidly.
   E. All effects of radiation also occur naturally, so expected rates must be compared with actual rates to find abnormalities.

II. Acute radiation syndrome in humans begins after the reception of a whole-body absorbed dose of 1 Gy (100 rad) or more delivered over a short period of time.
   A. Doses sufficient to cause acute radiation syndrome do not occur during modern diagnostic radiation procedures.
   B. Acute radiation syndrome normally results from accidents or the use of nuclear weapons.
   C. Acute radiation syndrome occurs only when the entire body is exposed, not simply when parts of the body receive high doses.
   D. Acute radiation syndrome symptoms include nausea, blood disorders, intestinal disorders, fever, fatigue, lowered sperm count, sterility in both sexes (temporary and permanent), cardiovascular system damage, central nervous system damage, and skin shedding.
   E. Acute radiation syndrome manifests itself in four major states.
      1. The prodromal stage occurs within a few hours after a whole-body absorbed dose of 1 Gy (100 rad) or more and can last up to several days.
      2. The latent stage does not have symptoms. This may last about a week.
      3. In the manifest illness stage, patients experience a wide range of visible symptoms, generally more severe than in the prodromal stage.
      4. The final stage is recovery or death.
   F. The three predictable biologic effects of acute radiation syndrome are hematopoietic syndrome, gastrointestinal syndrome, and cerebrovascular syndrome.

III. Hematopoietic syndrome (or bone marrow syndrome) can occur when humans receive a whole-body absorbed dose of about 1 to 10 Gy (100 to 1000 rad).

   A. With doses below 1 Gy (100 rad), bone marrow generally can recover within a few weeks.

   B. With doses above 10 Gy (1000 rad), bone marrow is severely damaged or destroyed, so recovery can be lengthy.

   C. Symptoms of hematopoietic syndrome include severe nausea, vomiting, diarrhea, and leukopenia.

   D. The radiosensitivity of cells differs at different stages of cell maturation.

      1. Immature blood cells are more radiosensitive than mature blood cells.

      2. Lymphocytes (a type of white blood cell) are the most radiosensitive blood cells in the human body.

      3. Mature red blood cells are the least radiosensitive of all blood cells.

      4. Generally, blood cells with longer lives are less radiosensitive.

   E. White blood cells include lymphocytes, granulocytes (neutrophilic and eosinophilic), and platelets (or thrombocytes).

      1. Damage to lymphocytes and granulocytes lowers the body's resistance to disease.

      2. Long-lived platelets (about 30 days) are relatively resistant to radiation damage, though they can be lessened by a dose of ionizing radiation greater than 0.5 Gy (50 rad).

   F. Numerous studies indicate chromosome aberrations in circulating lymphocytes that received radiation doses within the diagnostic range.

   G. Blood tests can help identify radiotherapy patients with lowered blood count; antibiotics can help counteract a lowered red blood cell count.

IV. Gastrointestinal syndrome begins with a threshold whole-body absorbed dose of about 6 Gy (600 rad) and peaks after a dose of 10 Gy (1000 rad).

   A. Most patients exposed to a whole-body dose of 6 to 10 Gy (600 to 1000 rads) do not survive more than 10 days.

   B. Symptoms of gastrointestinal syndrome include severe nausea, vomiting, and prolonged diarrhea. Other symptoms may include fever, fatigue, anemia, leukopenia, hemorrhage, electrolytic imbalance, and emaciation.

   C. Death from gastrointestinal syndrome occurs when the immature cells of the epithelial lining are killed by radiation and are not replaced.

      1. Radiation kills the crypt cells of Lieberkühn, which replace the villi cells on the intestinal lining.

      2. With the intestinal membrane exposed, fluids can pass through, resulting in an electrolytic imbalance.

V. Cerebrovascular syndrome occurs at doses above 50 Gy (5000 rad).

   A. Most patients exposed to a whole-body absorbed dose of 50 Gy (5000 rad) die in several hours to several days.

      1. The prodromal stage can begin within minutes.

      2. The latent stage can occur within hours but lasts only for 12 hours.

3. Symptoms of the manifest stage become increasingly severe.
4. Death results from failure of the central nervous and cardiovascular systems.

B. Symptoms of cerebrovascular syndrome include excessive nervousness, confusion, severe nausea, vomiting, diarrhea, loss of vision, a burning sensation of the skin, and loss of consciousness. Other symptoms may include disorientation, convulsive seizures, electrolytic imbalance, meningitis, prostration, and respiratory distress.

VI. Radiation effects on the embryo-fetus mirror the effects of radiation on cells.

A. The embryo-fetus is more sensitive to radiation than either children or adults.

B. Sensitivity of an embryo-fetus to radiation declines with maturity.
1. The most dangerous exposure time is the first trimester, between the second and eighth weeks of gestation, when the embryo-fetus contains a large number of stem cells, which are extremely radiosensitive.
2. Radiation exposure during the first 2 weeks is more likely to cause spontaneous abortion than future illness.

C. The Oxford Study explored the increased incidence of leukemia among children exposed to radiation in utero.

VII. LD 50/30 specifies the whole-body radiation dose at which 50% of the individuals exposed would die within 30 days.

A. Humans are not expected to die at doses less than 1 Gy (100 rad).

B. In humans, LD 50/30 occurs at 3 Gy (300 rad).

C. Generally, humans are not expected to survive doses above 6 Gy (600 rad).

D. Humans are much more radiosensitive than other animals.

E. Measurements other than LD 50/30—such as LD 50/60, LD 100/60, and LD 10/30—are sometimes used.

F. Mean survival time reflects the decrease in the time between exposure and death that usually results from increased radiation doses.

Review

Fill in the blank with the appropriate word or phrase. The answers are at the end of this module.

1. All early and late somatic and genetic radiation damage—from radiation skin burns to organ damage—can be traced to _____ radiation effect.

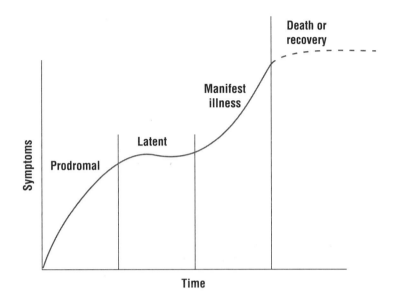

2. Understanding the dangers of high levels of radiation can help radiographers understand the _____.

3. Every radiation dose-response relationship is either _____ or _____ and _____ or _____.

DOSE-RESPONSE RELATIONSHIPS

4. The _____ nonthreshold curve shows that as the radiation dose increases, the response increases in an increasingly rapid manner.

5. The nonthreshold dose-response relationship means that _____ radiation can cause _____ response.

6. Name the four stages of acute radiation syndrome: _____, _____ period, _____ illness, and _____ or _____.

7. Early or acute somatic effects of radiation are generally the result of _____ or _____.

8. Death or recovery from acute radiation syndrome depends on _____.

9. The severity of symptoms of acute radiation are most closely related to the _____ and the _____ involved.

10. Name the three primary dose-related forms of acute radiation syndrome related to whole-body irradiation: _____, _____, and _____.

11. Different blood cells have different levels of _____.

12. The four primary types of blood cells are _____ blood cells, two types of _____ blood cells, and _____ cells.

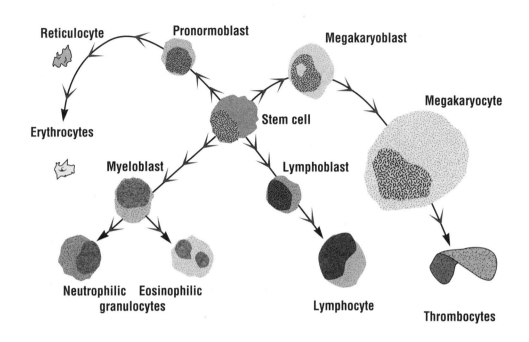

13. Before blood cells mature, they go through a _____ stage in the bone marrow.

14. Because of their relatively long life, mature red blood cells have _____ resistance to ionizing radiation.

15. A unique feature of red blood cells is the absence of a _____.

16. Each type of white blood cell has its own _____ and level of _____.

17. The high radiosensitivity of leukocytes, or _____ blood cells, is due to their _____ life.

18. _____ and _____ are the two types of granulocyte cells.

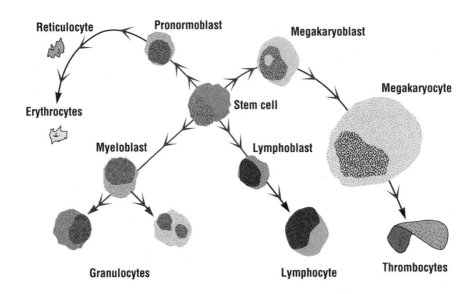

19. Platelet cells, also called _____, allow blood _____ and help control _____.

20. At a radiation dose of 1 Gy (100 rad), the blood count will begin to _____.

21. Common symptoms of hematopoietic and gastrointestinal syndromes include _____, _____, and _____.

22. Severe nausea, vomiting, diarrhea, nervousness, confusion, and a loss of vision are symptoms of _____ syndrome.

23. As an embryo-fetus ages, its sensitivity to ionizing radiation _____.

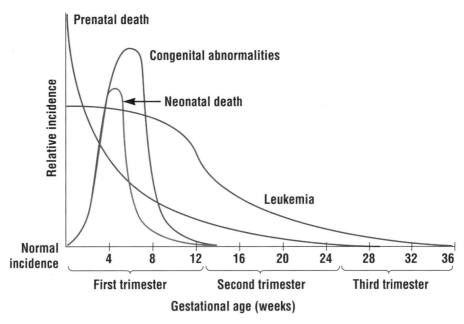

IN UTERO EFFECTS OF RADIATION AT 2 Gy (200 rad)

24. High doses of radiation can produce biologic effects that are _____ to biologic effects that occur naturally.

25. The embryo-fetus is particularly sensitive to radiation exposure during the first trimester because of the large number of _____ cells.

26. The most common effect of radiation exposure to an embryo-fetus during the first 2 weeks of the first trimester is _____.

27. LD 50/30 for humans is reached at a dose of _____.

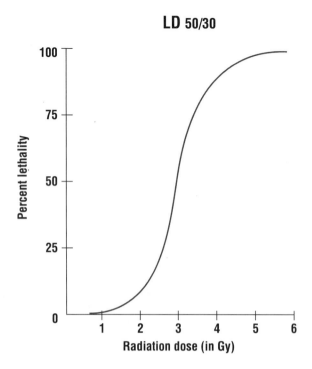

Learning Quiz

Some of the following learning questions are similar to the interactive exercises found in the CD-ROM version of this module operated in the "Student Mode." Please provide the best possible short answer. The answers are at the end of this module.

1. What are the two reasons scientists study the effects of high doses of radiation on humans? Why is it difficult to gather this information?

2. Why are patients with low white blood cell counts more susceptible to infections? How long does it take patients to recover from damage to white blood cells by radiation?

3. Describe how ionizing radiation damages the epithelial lining. What can result from this damage?

Applications

The following questions ask you to apply the knowledge you have gained from this module. Please provide the best possible answer. The answers are at the end of this module.

1. What do scientists hope to learn by studying radiation dose-response relationships?

2. Explain why it is often difficult to determine the true genetic effects of radiation exposure. How do scientists determine what effects to attribute to radiation?

3. Why are patients who are being treated with radiation therapy tested for drops in blood count?

4. Explain why physicians use antibiotics to counteract a lowered white blood cell count.

5. How can the understanding of the radiosensitivity of cells be applied to the radiosensitivity of an embryo-fetus?

6. Summarize the Oxford Study. How are the conclusions of this study controversial?

7. How would you advise a pregnant woman who works in an environment where she could face exposure to radiation?

Posttest

Circle the best answer for each of the following questions. Your instructor has the correct answers.

1. What is the effect of radiation in a threshold dose-response relationship?
   a. There is no effect.
   b. The severity of radiation damage is limited, regardless of the dose.
   c. Radiation response occurs at a specific threshold dose.
   d. A response to radiation will occur with any size dose.

2. What is the characteristic response of the human body to low levels of radiation?
   a. Linear nonthreshold
   b. Linear-quadratic nonthreshold
   c. Causes increasingly rapid response with increased dose
   d. All of the above
   e. None of the above

3. What is the extra measure of caution built into diagnostic radiation protection standards?
   a. Assume biologic response is directly proportional to increased dose.
   b. Assume biologic response is independent of dose.
   c. Remain below any known threshold.
   d. Keep dose to 50% of any known threshold.

4. What is an early, or acute, effect of radiation exposure?
   a. Genetic damage manifested in future generations
   b. Long-term damage detected months or years after exposure
   c. Multiple treatments in a short time period
   d. Identifiable biologic response to radiation within minutes, hours, days or weeks of the exposure

5. How long after whole-body exposure to a dose of 1 Gy (100 rad) does the prodromal stage of acute radiation syndrome begin?
   a. 3 to 5 days
   b. Generally within 1 month
   c. Within hours
   d. Seconds to minutes

6. What are the symptoms of the latent stage of acute radiation syndrome?
   a. Nausea, vomiting, diarrhea, fatigue, and an abnormal decrease in white blood cells
   b. Cardiovascular system failure
   c. Central nervous system and cardiovascular system failure
   d. No symptoms

7. What type of cancer has increased dramatically in children exposed to radiation from the Chernobyl nuclear power plant accident?
   a. Skin
   b. Lung
   c. Thyroid
   d. Breast
   e. Lymph node

8. What is the function of the hematopoietic system?
   a. Filters toxins from the blood
   b. Creates protein
   c. Manufactures the various types of cells in blood
   d. Manufactures bone marrow

9. At what dose does hematopoietic syndrome begin?
   a. 1 Gy (100 rad)
   b. 10 Gy (1000 rad)
   c. 0.1 Gy (10 rad)
   d. 100 Gy (10,000 rad)

10. What generally happens to bone marrow when it is exposed to a radiation dose of less than 1 Gy (100 rad)?
    a. Short-term damage, with recovery within a few weeks
    b. Permanent damage
    c. Severe long-term loss of stem cells
    d. No effect

11. What are the most radiosensitive blood cells in the human body?
    a. Immature red blood cells
    b. Immature platelet blood cells
    c. Mature red blood cells
    d. Lymphocytes

12. What blood cells are responsible for transporting oxygen and carbon dioxide throughout the body?
    a. Platelets
    b. White blood cells
    c. Red blood cells
    d. Stem cells

13. What is the approximate dose threshold for damage to leukocytes, or white blood cells?
    a. 25 Gy (2500 rad)
    b. 0.25 Gy (25 rad)
    c. 0.025 Gy (2.5 rad)
    d. 2.5 Gy (250 rad)

14. What blood cells produce antibodies to protect the body from disease?
    a. Lymphocytes
    b. Erythrocytes
    c. Granulocytes
    d. Neutrophils

15. How does the reaction of granulocyte cells to radiation differ from that of other blood cells?
    a. Granulocyte cells are unaffected by radiation.
    b. Radiation initiates rapid growth of granulocyte cells.
    c. Granulocyte cells increase sharply in number and then rapidly decrease.
    d. Radiation destroys all granulocyte cells.

16. At approximately what dose are platelet cells affected by ionizing radiation?
    a. 0.05 Gy (5 rad)
    b. 5 Gy (500 rad)
    c. 1.5 Gy (150 rad)
    d. 0.5 Gy (50 rad)

17. What is the greatest infection risk to patients with acute radiation syndrome?
    a. Other individuals
    b. Food poisoning
    c. Outside germs
    d. Bacteria and antigens in the body

18. Approximately how long does bone marrow take to recover after whole-body exposure to a radiation dose less than 1 Gy (100 rad)?
    a. Several hours
    b. Several days
    c. Weeks to months
    d. Years

19. What occurs when the cells lining the intestinal tract—villi—are damaged?
    a. The cells will absorb digested nutrients into the bloodstream.
    b. Homeostasis will be impaired.
    c. Electrolyte imbalances will occur.
    d. All of the above
    e. Answers (a) and (c) only

20. At what whole-body radiation dose does gastrointestinal syndrome begin?
    a. 0.10 Gy (10 rad)
    b. 1 Gy (100 rad)
    c. 6 Gy (600 rad)
    d. 10 Gy (1000 rad)

21. What is the length of time between radiation exposure and death from cerebrovascular syndrome?
    a. 1 to 15 minutes
    b. About a week
    c. From hours up to 2 or 3 days
    d. Roughly a month

22. What cells in the brain are critical to the body's communication system?
    a. Red blood cells
    b. Nerve cells
    c. Crypt cells of Lieberkühn
    d. White blood cells
    e. All of the above

23. What causes death in cerebrovascular syndrome?
    a. Damage to small blood vessels
    b. Hemorrhaging in the brain
    c. Elevated fluid content in the brain
    d. Elevated intracranial pressure
    e. All of the above

24. What impact does exposure to ionizing radiation have on naturally occurring genetic effects?
    a. There is no effect.
    b. Radiation exposure decreases the likelihood of these genetic effects.
    c. Radiation exposure increases the likelihood of naturally occurring genetic effects.
    d. The effect is not known.

25. What is the most dangerous time for an embryo-fetus to be exposed to ionizing radiation?
    a. During labor
    b. During the third trimester
    c. During the second trimester
    d. During the first trimester
    e. None of the above

26. At what radiation dose is an embryo-fetus expected to suffer massive damage from ionizing radiation?
    a. 0.1 Gy (10 rad)
    b. 0.01 Gy (1 rad)
    c. 2 Gy (200 rad)
    d. 0.2 Gy (20 rad)

27. What is the maximum recommended radiation exposure per month for individuals in radiation occupations?
    a. Less than 0.5 Sv (0.05 rem)
    b. Less than 0.3 Gy (30 rad)
    c. More than 5 Sv (0.5 rem)
    d. 5 Gy (500 rad)

28. Above what dose of radiation are no survivors expected?
    a. 1 Gy (100 rad)
    b. 3 Gy (300 rad)
    c. 4 Gy (400 rad)
    d. 6 Gy (600 rad)

29. What is the LD for the whole-body radiation dose at which 50% of the individuals exposed would die within 60 days?
    a. LD 60/50
    b. LD 30/60
    c. LD 50/30
    d. LD 50/60

30. How does an individual's size affect sensitivity to whole-body radiation exposure?
    a. Size has no effect.
    b. Radiosensitivity increases with body-size increase.
    c. Radiosensitivity decreases slightly with body-size increase.
    d. Radiosensitivity decreases dramatically with body-size increase.
    e. None of the above

Answer Key

Answers to Pretest

1. c

2. a

3. d

4. b

5. d

6. c

7. a

8. d

9. b

10. d

Answers to Review

1. Cellular
2. Dangers at low levels
3. Linear, nonlinear, threshold, nonthreshold
4. Linear-quadratic
5. Any, some
6. Prodromal, latent, manifest, recovery, death
7. Accidents, nuclear war
8. The amount of damage sustained by the body
9. Dose, individual
10. Hematopoietic or bone marrow syndrome, gastrointestinal syndrome, cerebrovascular syndrome
11. Radiosensitivity
12. Red, white, platelet
13. Transition
14. Increased
15. Nucleus
16. Function, radiosensitivity
17. White, short
18. Neutrophilic, eosinophilic
19. Thrombocytes, clotting, hemorrhaging
20. Drop
21. Nausea, vomiting, diarrhea
22. Cerebrovascular
23. Declines

24. Identical

25. Stem

26. Death by spontaneous abortion

27. 3 Gy (300 rad)

Answers to Learning Quiz

1. Scientists study the effects of high doses of radiation on humans for two primary reasons: (1) to improve medical care to the victims of high doses of radiation and (2) to learn what effect low levels of radiation may have on the human body by extrapolating the effects of high doses. This research is difficult because high doses generally occur only as a result of an accident (such as the Chernobyl nuclear power plant disaster) or war (such as the atomic bombing of Japan).

2. Lymphocytes, which produce antibodies to protect the body from disease, are the body's main disease defense. Lymphocytes also are the most radiosensitive of the white blood cells. Consequently, patients with a low lymphocyte count are more susceptible to infections than patients with a normal lymphocyte count. Depending on the damage by ionizing radiation, recovery after exposure can take from a few days to several months.

3. Although radiation exposure may not seriously damage the functioning cells of the epithelial lining, radiation exposure can kill the crypt cells of Lieberkühn, which provide new cells. With no new cells being produced, the villi will wear away and the intestinal membrane will become exposed. With the intestinal membrane exposed, fluids can pass through it, resulting in an electrolyte imbalance.

Answers to Applications

1. Scientists study radiation dose-response relationships—that is, the effects of radiation observed in relation to the dose of radiation received by humans—for two primary reasons: (1) to understand how to apply radiation as a therapeutic treatment for malignant diseases and (2) to better understand the biologic effects of low-dose irradiation.

2. The genetic effects of radiation exposure are difficult to quantify because all of these effects also occur naturally. To identify effects actually caused by radiation, scientists compare the predicted rate of natural occurrence of an abnormality with the rate found in individuals exposed to radiation.

3. A therapeutic dose of ionizing radiation causes a decrease in the blood count. Patients' blood counts are monitored, usually weekly or biweekly, to determine whether the platelet count is adequate.

4. White blood cells are the body's primary protection against infection. If these cells are reduced in number—such as from radiation therapy—the risk to infection increases. Antibiotics help counteract the effects of the lowered white blood cell count.

5. An embryo-fetus progresses through the various stages of cell development. As with cells, the radiosensitivity of an embryo-fetus is greatest when the rate of cell reproduction is highest, and radiosensitivity decreases with age.

6. The Oxford Study examined the increased incidence of leukemia among children exposed to diagnostic radiation in utero. Scientists have used this data to develop a table of relative risk. The conclusions of the study have been challenged because of the possibility that some factor or factors other than diagnostic radiation caused the increased incidence of leukemia.

7. Any worker who risks exposure to unplanned ionizing radiation and becomes pregnant should discuss safety precautions with someone qualified to assess radiation safety. If needed, the worker's schedule or assignment must be altered.

Genetic Effects

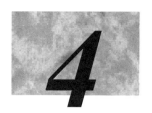

Self-Assessment Pretest

Before you begin to work through the Review, Learning Quiz, and Application exercises, use this pretest to assess your knowledge of the material in this module. Circle the best answer for each of the following questions. The answers are at the end of this module.

1. What is the most common result of interaction between an x-ray photon and a molecule in the body?
   a. Cell death
   b. Patient death
   c. Permanent chromosome damage
   d. Late-effect genetic damage
   e. Insignificant cell or water molecule damage

2. What is the primary cause of cell damage at low doses of ionizing radiation?
   a. Cross-linking
   b. Main-chain scission
   c. Point lesions
   d. Decreased cell fluid viscosity

3. What is late-effect genetic damage?
   a. Damage to a somatic cell
   b. Damage to a lymphocyte
   c. Damage to DNA that is not expressed until late in an exposed individual's life
   d. Damage—not seen for generations—to a DNA molecule in a germ cell of an adult

4. Which of the following statements accurately characterizes human genes?
   a. Every human cell contains the same genes.
   b. Every human cell contains different genes.
   c. All male cells contain the same genes, whereas all female cells do not contain the same genes.
   d. Every human cell contains 1 of 23 combinations of genes.
   e. Every human cell contains 1 of 46 combinations of genes.

5. What condition must exist for a recessive gene mutation to be expressed?
   a. The mutated gene must be paired with a dominant mutation.
   b. The mutated gene must be present in both parents.
   c. The mutated gene must be present in only one parent.
   d. The mutated gene must be dominant.

Module 4: Genetic Effects   73

6. What is the impact of diagnostic radiography on changes in the number of chromosomes?
   a. Very high risk of changes
   b. Seldom causes changes
   c. Never causes changes
   d. Seldom causes changes in females; sometimes causes changes in males

7. What results when the child of a person with reciprocal translocation aberration receives only one of the rearranged chromosome fragments?
   a. Possible embryonic death
   b. Possible physical abnormalities
   c. Possible mental abnormalities
   d. Genetically unbalanced cells
   e. Any of the above

8. What is the genetic risk of radiation exposure resulting from both a known radiation exposure and naturally occurring risk called?
   a. Doubling risk
   b. Relative risk
   c. Absolute risk
   d. Reciprocal translocation risk
   e. None of the above

9. To minimize the risk of passing on a genetic mutation, conception should be postponed for how long after the possible irradiation of sperm?
   a. 1 week to 10 days
   b. 1 month
   c. Several months
   d. 6 to 10 years

10. How long should female patients wait to conceive after an ovarian dose of 0.10 Gy (10 rad)?
    a. 1 menstrual cycle
    b. 1 month
    c. 1 year
    d. Several months

Key Terms

Before continuing, be sure you can define the following key terms.

Absolute risk: The total risk of genetic mutation appearing in a certain population.

Autosomes: The 22 pairs of human chromosomes that are not sex chromosomes.

Cross-linking: The effect of ionizing radiation on DNA and other macromolecules after main-chain scission, which causes spurlike molecules on a molecular chain to stick to the molecular chain or to other molecules.

Dicentric chromosome: The formation resulting when two adjacent chromosomes that are struck in the G_1 phase join during the S phase of interphase; dicentric chromosomes generally result in cell death.

Dominant gene mutation: The most common type of gene mutation; expressed in the first generation; examples include Huntington's chorea, polydactyly, and retinoblastoma.

Dose-rate effect: The decrease in mutations as a radiation dose is given over a longer period of time.

Down syndrome: A chromosomal aberration caused by the presence of an extra chromosome 21.

Doubling dose: The dose of ionizing radiation that would produce twice the frequency of genetic mutations as expected to occur naturally.

Gene: A specific section of the DNA double helix that contains a specific sequence of nitrogenous organic bases; the basic unit of heredity.

Genetic code: An individual's unique genetic makeup, as determined by the sequence of the nitrogenous organic bases in each gene.

Genetic effects: The effects of ionizing radiation on future generations.

Genetics: The study of the inheritance of characteristics.

Interphase: The period when a cell is growing and copying chromosomes in preparation for cell division.

Karyotyping: Using a microscope to identify and map genes.

Late-effect genetic damage: Genetic damage from exposure to ionizing radiation that may not be seen for generations.

Main-chain scission: The condition resulting from breakage of the thread or backbone of a long-chain molecule.

Molecular lesion: Damage resulting when the chemical bonds of molecules are disrupted; also known as *point lesion*.

Multi-hit chromosome aberrations: A single chromosome struck more than once.

Point lesion: Damage resulting damage when the chemical bonds of molecules are disrupted; also known as molecular lesion.

Recessive gene mutation: Both genes must be recessive for a recessive gene mutation to be expressed, unless sex-linked; less common than dominant gene mutations, recessive gene mutations are traced to more than 1100 diseases; examples include cystic fibrosis, sickle-cell anemia, and Tay-Sachs disease.

Reciprocal translocation aberration: A multi-hit aberration in which the tops of adjacent chromosomes are broken and the resulting fragments attach to one another; the most common form of radiation-induced chromosomal abnormalities, reciprocal translocation aberrations may not necessarily result in cell death.

Relative risk: Refers to the increased risk of genetic mutation due to exposure to ionizing radiation; the ratio of the risk of mutations resulting from ionizing radiation to the naturally occurring risk.

Ring formation: The formation that results when the ends of a severed chromosome join, forming a ring; generally results in cell death.

Sex-linked gene mutation: Recessive gene mutation found on the X chromosome (that is, expressed without a complementary gene); expressed in males because there is no matching gene in the male's Y chromosome; examples include color blindness, hemophilia, and a form of muscular dystrophy.

Single-hit chromosome aberration: One chromosome struck in one location.

Topical Outline

The following material is covered in this module.

I. The interactions of x-ray photons with atoms composing the molecules in the human body can cause biologic changes that result in genetic effects.
   A. The interactions of x-ray photons with atoms and molecules in the body usually results in insignificant damage.
   B. The irradiation of DNA or any other macromolecule can have three major effects.
      1. Main-chain scission occurs when the thread or backbone of the long-chain molecule breaks.
      2. After main-chain scission, macromolecules can cross-link via sticky, spurlike molecules that extend from the main macromolecule chain.
      3. Molecular or point lesions occur when the chemical bonds of a molecule are disrupted.
   C. Cells often can repair themselves when main-chain scission, cross-linking, and point lesions occur.
   D. Damage to DNA can cause cell death and can change metabolic activity, causing cells to reproduce more rapidly than normally.
   E. Damaged DNA can result in late-effect genetic damage, which means the damage may not be seen for generations.
   F. Three ways in which DNA damage affects chromosomes are terminal deletion, dicentric formation, and ring formation.
II. Understanding the genetic effects of ionizing radiation requires an understanding of genetics.
   A. Genetics refers to the study of the inheritance of characteristics.
      1. Inherited characteristics include molecular and cellular formations.
      2. Inherited characteristics extend to physiological and behavioral traits.
   B. Genes are sections of the DNA double helix.

1. Every gene contains a sequence of nitrogenous organic bases.
2. The sequence of bases determines an individual's genetic code.
C. All human cells contain the same genes.
D. The function of a particular cell is determined by the activity of the genes in that cell.
E. 22 pairs of chromosomes in humans are autosomes; 1 pair consists of sex chromosomes.
    1. All cells in males contain a large X chromosome and a small Y chromosome.
    2. All cells in females contain two X chromosomes and no Y chromosomes.
F. An individual inherits half of his or her genes from each parent.
G. Genes can be dominant or recessive.
    1. A dominant gene is expressed when matched with a recessive gene.
    2. A recessive gene expresses itself only when matched with another recessive gene.
    3. Dominant gene mutations and sex-linked gene mutations will appear in the first generation of males.

III. Genetic mutations can be dominant, recessive, or sex-linked.
    A. Dominant gene mutations, which are expressed in the first generation, are the most common genetic mutations.
    B. Most radiation-induced genetic mutations—the second most common mutations—are recessive.
        1. Recessive mutations must be present from both parents to be expressed.
        2. Radiation-induced genetic mutations cannot be differentiated from other genetic mutations.
        3. Scientists theorize that radiation-induced mutations will increase as more and more people are exposed to ionizing radiation.
    C. Sex-linked gene mutations are the least common genetic mutation.
    D. Individuals who work with ionizing radiation must take a conservative approach to genetic mutations, even at low energy levels.

IV. Genetic disorders resulting from chromosomal aberrations also are affected by ionizing radiation.
    A. Chromosomal aberrations generally result from having too few or too many chromosomes.
        1. Down syndrome—possibly the best known chromosomal aberration—results from the presence of an extra chromosome 21.
        2. A large percentage of spontaneous abortions are attributed to chromosomal disorders.
    B. Radiation—particularly at the diagnostic level—rarely causes changes in the number of chromosomes.
        1. When both ends of a severed chromosome attach, a ring formation occurs.

2. When two adjacent chromosomes are struck during the G_1 phase and then join during the S phase of interphase, a dicentric chromosome forms.

3. A reciprocal translocation aberration occurs when the tops of adjacent chromosomes are severed but the resulting fragments attach to one another, and thus all or most of the genetic material is saved.

C. The chance that ionizing radiation will break or damage a chromosome depends on a number of factors, including the stage of cell life and the number of times the chromosome is struck by x-ray photons.

1. Chromosome aberrations occur when a cell is irradiated in the early stage of interphase.

2. Multi-hit chromosome aberrations can result in the severing of both ends of a chromosome, the formation of a ring, and cell death.

3. Multi-hit chromosome aberrations that are reciprocal translocation aberrations may not be lethal.

D. The radiation dose affects the occurrence of single- and multi-hit aberrations.

V. Understanding the risk estimates of radiation-induced genetic mutations is important for anyone working with ionizing radiation.

A. The risk estimates of radiation-induced genetic mutations are complex.

1. Radiation-induced genetic mutations are identical to naturally occurring mutations.

2. Radiation-induced genetic mutations are extremely rare.

3. Detecting radiation-induced genetic mutations requires a huge population sample.

4. Little data on radiation-induced mutation in humans are available.

B. Scientists use a number of methods to assess the genetic risk of radiation exposure.

1. Absolute risk combines the risk of a known radiation exposure with the naturally occurring risk.

2. Relative risk considers the increased risk due to exposure to ionizing radiation.

3. The doubling dose identifies the dose of ionizing radiation that would produce twice the frequency of mutations that naturally occurs.

C. The most important risk factor is sex, with males being more sensitive to radiation than females.

VI. The results of genetic radiation research reflect the complexity of this topic.

A. H. J. Muller studied the effects of ionizing radiation on fruit flies.

B. The Russells experimented with mice.

1. Different mutations have different radiosensitivities.

2. The dose rate effect reflects the decrease in mutations as a radiation dose is given over a longer period of time, as a result of the ability of cells to repair themselves.

C. Both studies make a connection between radiation and genetic mutation, although these conclusions have not been verified.

Review

Fill in the blank with the appropriate word or phrase. The answers are at the end of this module.

1. All damage to molecules from ionizing radiation begins with an interaction between a single x-ray _____ and an atom.

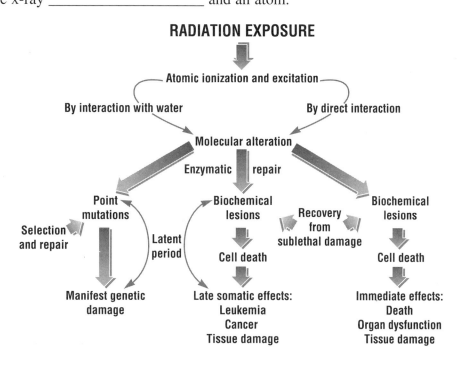

2. Name three major effects that can occur when DNA or other macromolecules are irradiated: _____, _____, and _____.

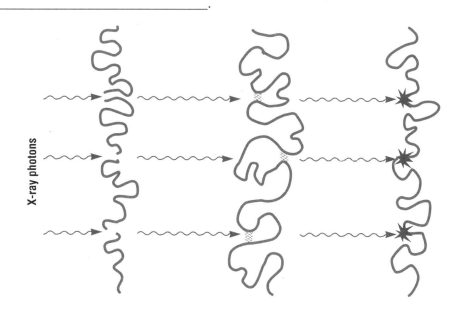

3. A main-chain scission can occur if one or both of the side rails of the DNA or RNA _____ are cut.

4. In cross-linking, broken molecules can attach to other _____, to new _____, or to _____.

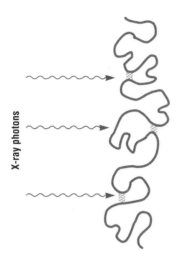

5. Point lesions can occur as a _____ or _____ effect of irradiation.

6. When a point lesion occurs in a stem cell or reproductive cell, some nitrogenous organic _____ in the DNA _____ may be missing. These missing elements control aspects of cell _____.

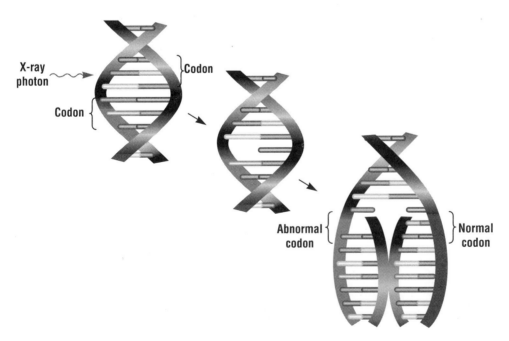

80   Module 4: Genetic Effects

7. The damage caused by main-chain scission, cross-linking, and point lesions is not always permanent because of the cells' ability to _____ themselves.

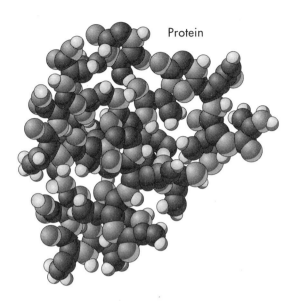

8. Name three types of chromosome damage: _____ deletion, _____ formation, and _____ formation.

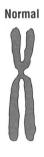

Normal chromosome

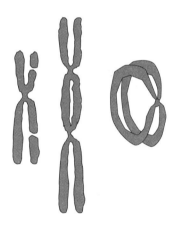

Abnormal chromosomes

9. Minor radiation-induced changes in DNA can result in _____ genetic abnormalities.

Module 4: Genetic Effects 81

10. An individual's genetic code is carried in the _____, which consist of DNA _____.

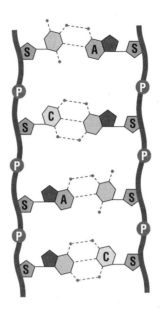

11. Each gene contains a certain sequence of _____ bases. An individual's unique genetic code is determined by the _____ of these bases.

12. The combination of a variety of genes determines an individual's _____.

13. All individuals inherit _____ of their genes from their father and _____ from their mother. The genes are either _____ or _____.

14. A recessive gene expresses itself when matched with _____.

15. Because they are not unique, radiation-induced genetic mutations cannot be distinguished from _____.

16. The natural occurrence of chromosomal aberrations normally results from having too _____ or too _____ chromosomes. Many spontaneous _____ are attributed to chromosomal disorders.

82 Module 4: Genetic Effects

17. The two key factors in how a cell is affected by ionizing radiation are the stage of the cell's _____ and the number of _____ by x-ray photons.

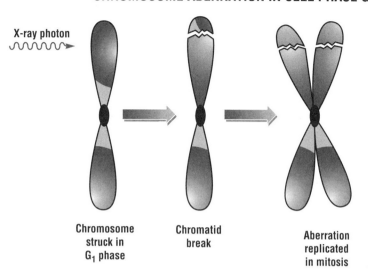

CHROMOSOME ABERRATION IN CELL PHASE G₁

Chromosome struck in G₁ phase → Chromatid break → Aberration replicated in mitosis

18. A ring formation is the result of a _____ chromosome aberration.

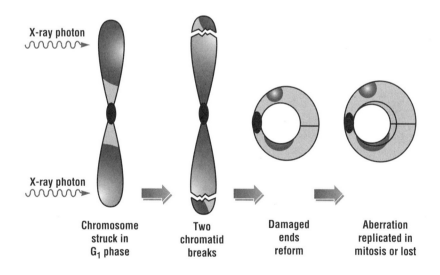

Chromosome struck in G₁ phase → Two chromatid breaks → Damaged ends reform → Aberration replicated in mitosis or lost

Module 4: Genetic Effects 83

19. Radiation-induced chromosomal aberrations usually result from _____.

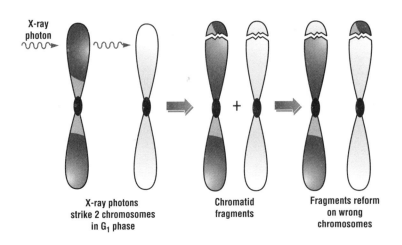

20. Translocation of chromatid fragments may not be harmful as long as most rearranged _____ remain and contain the complete set of _____.

21. The _____ dose directly affects the likelihood of single- and multi-hit aberrations.

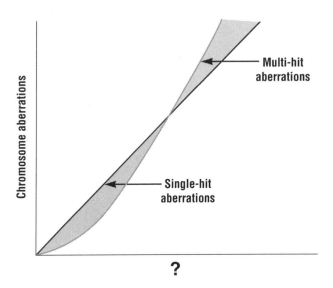

22. Multi-hit aberrations are characterized by a nonlinear dose-response relationship, because their increase is not _____ to the radiation dose.

84 Module 4: Genetic Effects

23. The assessment of absolute risk assumes a _____ dose-response relationship.

24. The doubling dose for humans is _____ Gy or _____ rad.

25. A low doubling rate for a certain genetic mutation means the radiosensitivity of that mutation is _____ (high/low).

26. Name the three areas related to children that scientists focused on when studying the survivors of the Hiroshima and Nagasaki bombings: _____, _____, and _____.

27. Most genetic mutations occur when sperm is _____, undergoes _____, and _____ an ovum.

28. Muller's studies of irradiated fruit flies revealed a _____, _____ dose-response relationship.

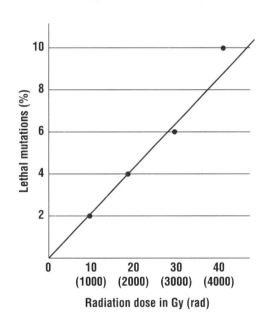

29. The Russells' megamouse study determined that genetic mutations could be induced by _____.

Module 4: Genetic Effects 85

30. The reproductive organs of _____ are more radiosensitive than

    _____ because of how cells are formed and mature.

Learning Quiz

Some of the following learning questions are similar to the interactive exercises found in the CD-ROM version of this module operated in the "Student Mode." Please provide the best possible short answer. The answers are at the end of this module.

1. Given that the genes in each human cell are the same, explain why there are different types of cells.

2. Explain why males have sex-linked genetic disorders that do not affect women. What implications can this have for male children of women?

Applications

The following questions ask you to apply the knowledge you have gained from this module. Please provide the best possible answer. The answers are at the end of this module.

1. How do researchers determine the degree of main-chain scission?

2. Explain how DNA macromolecules are damaged through indirect action of an x-ray photon.

3. Why do scientists use karyotyping to map genes? What is the importance of this work?

4. Why is the likelihood very low that a genetic mutation caused by low doses of ionizing radiation will express itself? Explain why scientists fear that this risk is increasing.

5. Explain why understanding radiation-induced genetic mutation is a challenge for scientists. Where does human radiation-exposure data come from?

Posttest

Circle the best answer for each of the following questions. Your instructor has the correct answers.

1. What causes main-chain scission?
   a. Cross-linking
   b. Molecular lesions
   c. Breakage in the thread or backbone of a long-chain molecule
   d. All of the above
   e. None of the above

2. What occurs when the spurlike molecules extending off a macromolecule chain attach to other parts of the chain or to other macromolecules?
   a. Cross-linking
   b. Point lesions
   c. Catabolized macromolecular lesions
   d. Main-chain scission

3. What is the effect of cross-linking?
   a. Broken molecules attach to other broken molecules.
   b. Broken molecules attach to themselves.
   c. Broken molecules attach to new molecules.
   d. All of the above
   e. Answers (a) and (c) only

4. When do molecular lesions or point lesions occur?
   a. During cross-linking
   b. When single chemical bonds of molecules are disrupted
   c. After main-chain scission
   d. When the DNA strand is broken
   e. All of the above

5. How does human tissue or an organ in the body survive high doses of ionizing radiation?
   a. Atrophy
   b. Repair of damaged cells
   c. Repopulation of lost cells
   d. All of the above
   e. Answers (b) and (c) only

6. What happens when the metabolic activity of cells changes?
   a. Cells reproduction ceases.
   b. Cells reproduce more rapidly.
   c. Cells atrophy.
   d. Cell fluid viscosity decreases.

7. Which of the following is *not* a nitrogenous organic base?
   a. Protein
   b. Adenine
   c. Guanine
   d. Thymine
   e. Cytosine

8. How many chromosomes do humans normally have?
   a. 23
   b. 46
   c. 46 pairs
   d. 92

9. How may human chromosomes are autosomes?
   a. 22
   b. 22 pairs
   c. 1 pair
   d. All chromosomes
   e. None of the above

10. What is the cell configuration in males?
    a. Large X chromosome and small Y chromosome
    b. Large Y chromosome and small X chromosome
    c. Two Y chromosomes and no X chromosomes
    d. Large X chromosome and large Y chromosome

11. Why are some gene mutations expressed without a complementary gene?
    a. Females have no X chromosome.
    b. Males have only one Y chromosome.
    c. Females have two Y chromosomes.
    d. Males have one X chromosome.

12. What happens to a recessive mutant gene when it is suppressed?
    a. It remains suppressed.
    b. It is no longer mutant.
    c. It disappears.
    d. It cannot be passed on.

13. What determines whether or not a mutated gene in the sperm or ovum is expressed in the following generation?
    a. Whether or not the gene is dominant
    b. Whether or not the gene is recessive
    c. Whether or not the gene is sex-linked
    d. All of the above
    e. None of the above

14. What is the characteristic of most radiation-induced genetic mutations?
    a. Dominant gene
    b. Recessive gene
    c. Sex-linked gene
    d. No difference
    e. None of the above

15. What chromosome aberration is most likely to result from ionizing radiation?
    a. Changes in the number of chromosomes in males
    b. Changes in the number of chromosomes in either sex
    c. Damaged or broken chromosomes
    d. Changes in the number or chromosomes in females

16. What is a single-hit chromosome aberration?
    a. Chromosome damage caused by a single x-ray photon
    b. Chromosome damage to a single chromosome caused by a single x-ray photon
    c. A single chromosome broken in one location
    d. All of the above

17. What can result when two adjacent chromosomes are struck in the G_1 phase?
    a. They can join during the S phase of interphase.
    b. A dicentric chromosome can be formed.
    c. A chromosome with two centromeres can be formed.
    d. A chromosome missing significant genetic material can be formed.
    e. Any of the above

18. What is the effect of reciprocal translocation on cell development?
    a. Normal cell development ceases.
    b. The cell generally dies quickly.
    c. Cell development often is not affected.
    d. Cell development proceeds much more slowly than it normally would.

19. How are single-hit aberrations characterized?
    a. They are produced with a linear, nonthreshold, dose-response relationship.
    b. They increase proportionally to the radiation dose.
    c. They occur at all doses of radiation.
    d. All of the above
    e. None of the above

20. When is relative risk a helpful tool for researchers?
    a. When precise data are available regarding radiation exposure
    b. When precise data are available regarding the naturally occurring risk of mutations
    c. When exact ionizing radiation doses are not known
    d. All of the above
    e. None of the above

21. What is the key factor in the risk of genetic mutation of ionizing radiation?
    a. Age
    b. Health
    c. Sex
    d. Race

22. What did H. J. Muller's study of irradiated fruit flies determine about genetic mutations?
    a. Radiation does not create new forms of mutations.
    b. Radiation does not change the quality of mutations.
    c. Radiation increases the frequency of mutations over.
    d. All of the above
    e. None of the above

Answer Key

Answers to Pretest

1. e
2. c
3. d
4. a
5. b
6. b
7. e
8. c
9. c
10. d

Answers to Review

1. Photon
2. Main-chain scission, cross-linking, molecular lesions or point lesions
3. Double helix
4. Broken molecules, molecules, themselves
5. Direct, indirect
6. Bases, strand, development or growth
7. Repair
8. Terminal, dicentric, ring
9. Important or major
10. Chromosomes, macromolecules

11. Nitrogenous organic, sequence

12. Characteristics

13. Half, half, dominant, recessive

14. Another recessive gene

15. Other genetic mutations

16. Few, many, abortions

17. Life, hits or strikes

18. Multi-hit

19. Reciprocal translocation

20. Chromosomes, genes

21. Radiation

22. Proportional

23. Linear

24. 0.5–2.5, 50–250

25. High

26. Severe pregnancy outcomes, death rate of children, sex chromosome abnormalities

27. Irradiated, mutation, fertilizes

28. Linear, nonthreshold

29. Ionizing radiation

30. Males, females

Answers to Learning Quiz

1. Although each human cell has the same genes, the actual function of the cell is determined by which genes are "turned on." Genes are used differently by different cells.

Module 4: Genetic Effects **93**

2. Unlike males, females always require a matching gene for genetic mutations because they have two X chromosomes. Thus, men have sex-linked genetic disorders that do not affect women. Women can pass on genetic disorders, however, which can then be expressed in male descendants.

Answers to Applications

1. Because the cytoplasm in a cell becomes thinner when main-chain scission occurs, the viscosity of fluid in the cell decreases. Researchers can determine the degree of main-chain scission by determining the change in viscosity.

2. When an x-ray photon interacts with a water molecule, a free radical can be formed. This free radical can migrate to another molecule (like DNA) and destroy the chemical bonds of that molecule or combine with molecules to form toxic substances. The result could be damage to a DNA macromolecule.

3. Using a microscope to identify and map genes—a process called karyotyping—enables scientists to compare an individual's genes with normal genes to uncover abnormal genes. By studying the genes from individuals with similar genetic abnormalities, scientists can determine what genes are causing the abnormality, which can help find cures for genetically based diseases. As with many diseases, early diagnosis is often critical in treatment.

4. Genetic mutations in general are rare. In addition, ionizing radiation is thought to be most closely associated with recessive mutations, which are not expressed unless both parents have the recessive gene. Unfortunately, however, as increasingly more people are exposed to ionizing radiation, the likelihood of both parents of an offspring having the same mutation is increasing.

5. Radiation-induced genetic mutations are identical to naturally occurring genetic mutations. In addition, they are extremely rare; thus huge sample sizes are required to detect small increases in genetic mutations resulting from radiation. Human data must be drawn from the bombing of Hiroshima and Nagasaki. Most risk studies are based on animal studies.

Somatic Effects

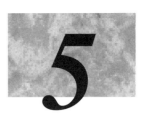

Self-Assessment Pretest

Before you begin to work through the Review, Learning Quiz, and Application exercises, use this pretest to assess your knowledge of the material in this module. Circle the best answer for each of the following questions. The answers are at the end of this module.

1. What is the time period for late somatic effects?
   a. Always late in the victim's lifetime
   b. Many generations after exposure to ionizing radiation
   c. Months, years, and decades after exposure to ionizing radiation
   d. Hours, days, and weeks after exposure to ionizing radiation

2. Approximately how many diseases are grouped under the term "cancer"?
   a. 1000
   b. 100
   c. 10
   d. 2

3. Which of the following is one of the most common sources of carcinogens?
   a. Occupational exposure to chemicals
   b. Environmental pollution
   c. Diagnostic radiography
   d. Chemicals in tobacco products

4. How is gene p53 different from other genes?
   a. It suppresses tumors.
   b. It is unable to suppress tumors.
   c. It suppresses and kills tumors.
   d. It cannot be damaged.

5. What is the latent period of solid tumors?
   a. 1 to 5 years
   b. 5 to 10 years
   c. 5 to 20 years
   d. 20 to 50 years

6. What is the probability of a woman developing breast cancer?
   a. 1 in 3
   b. 1 in 9
   c. 1 in 20
   d. 1 in 50
   e. 1 in 90

7. What is the number one cancer killer?
   a. Lung cancer
   b. Thyroid cancer
   c. Skin cancer
   d. Breast cancer
   e. Leukemia

8. What is the most common cause of skin cancer?
   a. Exposure to the sun
   b. Exposure to chemical carcinogens
   c. Radiation exposure
   d. Old age

9. What is the normal latent period for thyroid cancer?
   a. Less than a year
   b. 1 to 5 years
   c. 5 to 10 years
   d. 10 to 20 years
   e. 20 to 50 years

10. What characteristic makes lung cancer such a deadly disease?
    a. It strikes people when they are relatively young.
    b. It affects nonsmokers.
    c. It is one of the more difficult cancers to detect early.
    d. It can metastasize.

Key Terms

Before continuing, be sure you can define the following key terms.

Absolute risk: The total risk of malignancy appearing in a certain population; used when data on radiation doses is available; predicts that a specific number of excess malignancies will occur as a result of exposure.

Ann Arbor Series: A thyroid cancer study that consisted of individuals who had received radiation doses of 0.2 to 0.3 Gy (20 to 30 rad) to the thyroid gland shortly after birth for thymic enlargement due to infection.

BEIR Committee: Committee on the Biological Effects of Ionizing Radiation.

Carcinogenesis: The development of cancer.

Carcinogens: Cancer-causing agents.

Carcinomas: Solid tumors that start in the epithelial tissue; one of the two major categories of cancers.

Gene p53: Unlike other genes, gene p53 not only suppresses tumors but also kills them.

Gene amplification: The over-expression of a gene that occurs when there are extra copies of the proto-oncogene in a cell.

Late somatic effects: Effects such as malignancies that appear months, years, and decades after ionizing radiation has affected somatic cells.

Latent period: The period between the interaction with a cancer-causing agent and the expression of the cancer.

LET: Linear energy transfer. The amount of energy transferred on average by incident radiation to an object per unit of length of travel through the object.

Leukemia: Literally, "white blood"; a neoplastic overproduction of white blood cells.

Metastasize: To spread to other parts of the body.

Oncogenes: Genes that direct a cell to function abnormally.

Point mutations: The genetic mutation that results when a single base pair in the DNA strand is lost or changed.

Proto-oncogenes: The source of oncogenes; present in all mammalian cells, proto-oncogenes participate in normal cell growth.

Radon: A colorless, odorless, chemically inert, heavy radioactive gas; a decay product of uranium.

Reciprocal translocation: Fragments of one chromosome attaching to the fragments of another, possibly resulting in the alteration of some genetic information.

Relative risk: The percentage ratio of the risk of malignancy resulting from ionizing radiation to the naturally occurring risk; used to estimate late radiation effects on large populations without having any precise knowledge of their radiation dose.

Rochester Series: A thyroid cancer study that consisted of individuals who had received doses of about 3 Gy (300 rad) to the thyroid gland shortly after birth for thymic enlargement due to infection.

Rongelap Atoll Series: One thyroid cancer study that consisted of individuals who received a mean dose of radiation of 21 Gy (2100 rad) to the thyroid gland during childhood from atomic bomb testing.

Sarcomas: Cancers that begin in connective tissue; one of the two major categories of cancers.

Somatic cells: All the cells in the human body with the exception of germ cells.

Suppressor genes: Genes that suppress the replication of malignant cells.

Topical Outline

The following material is covered in this module.

I. Radiation-induced carcinogenesis involves cell damage and genetic mutation.
   A. The link between ionizing radiation and cancer was established in the early days of radiation research.
      1. Marie Curie and her daughter died of leukemia as a result of their work with radiation.
      2. X-ray dermatitis was a common condition of early researchers and radiologists.
   B. All cancer is characterized by the uncontrolled growth and spread of abnormal cells.
   C. Any human cell can become cancerous.
   D. Cancer is the end result of a series of events occurring within a cell, not a single event.
      1. The activation of oncogenes is one step.
         a. Oncogenes are formed from normal proto-oncogenes.
         b. Radiation can activate a proto-oncogene to produce a malignant cell through point mutation, chromosomal reciprocal translocation, and gene amplification.
      2. The loss of suppressor genes is another step.
         a. Suppressor genes suppress the replication of malignant cells.
         b. A loss of suppressor genes can result from ionizing radiation, cigarette smoking, chemical agents, and sunburn.
         c. Suppressor gene alteration generally results from point mutation.
         d. Much research into suppressor genes has involved gene p53.
      3. Other steps include inherited or activated gene mutations that increase susceptibility to becoming malignant.
   E. Cancers can either stay in one location or metastasize.
   F. Approximately 80% of cancers result from exposure to carcinogens.
      1. Chemicals and radiation are the primary types of carcinogens.
      2. Everyone comes in contact with carcinogens, both through occupational exposure and through lifestyle exposure.
      3. Most lung cancer is related to cigarette smoking.
      4. A cancer caused by chemicals is not different in physical appearance from the same cancer caused by ionizing radiation.
   G. Severity of cancer does not depend on the dose of ionizing radiation.
   H. Probability of cancer does depend on the dose of ionizing radiation.
   I. The latent period between exposure to ionizing radiation and expression of a cancer can last from months to many years.
      1. Leukemia has a relatively short latent period, often less than 10 years.

2. Solid tumors have a relatively long latent period, often 20 to 50 years.
J. The link between ionizing radiation and cancers explains the extensive personal protection procedures in radiography.

II. Scientists base risk assessment on data from populations that have received higher-than-normal doses of ionizing radiation.
   A. The Committee on the Biological Effects of Ionizing Radiation (BEIR Committee) directs many radiation risk studies.
   B. The risk of ionizing radiation exposure to patients, radiologists, and imaging personnel is considered to be extremely low.
      1. Protective measures lower the occupational risk of death to 1 in 100,000 for persons working in radiation-related occupations with exposure to 0.001 Gy (100 mrad).
      2. Any dose of ionizing radiation, regardless of how low, causes some increase in the risk of cancer.
   C. The normal expectation of cancer risk is higher among men than women.
   D. Cancer risk is related to age at the time of exposure.
   E. Researchers use two primary models to assess risk.
      1. Absolute risk is often used when data are available on radiation doses. This model predicts that a specific number of excess malignancies will occur as a result of exposure.
      2. Relative risk is usually used when information is not available on specific doses. This model predicts a percentage increase in incidence rather than a specific number of cases.
   F. The diagnostic benefits of radiography far outweigh any possible risk of radiation-induced cancer.

III. Different types of cancers are affected differently by ionizing radiation.
   A. Cancers are classified in more than 1000 ways in the laboratory.
   B. Cancers generally are grouped by their point of origin.
      1. Sarcomas begin in connective tissue, which forms bones, cartilage, muscle, fat, blood vessels, and the lymph system.
      2. Carcinomas are solid tumors that start in the epithelial tissue, which forms the skin and lining of most glands and organs.
   C. The most common cancer sites are the skin, lungs, female breasts, colon, rectum, uterus, blood-forming tissues, and the lymphatic system.
      1. Most skin cancer results from over-exposure to the sun.
      2. Lung cancer is one of the major cancer killers.
      3. About 1 in 9 women will develop breast cancer.
      4. Leukemias, cancers of the blood-forming tissues, are the most common cancer in children.
      5. Thyroid cancers have been related to ionizing radiation exposure in a number of studies.

Review

Fill in the blank with the appropriate word or phrase. The answers are at the end of this module.

1. Carcinogenesis involves cell _____ and genetic _____.

2. _____ and hereditary genetic _____ can result when cells are modified by irradiation.

3. The greater the radiation exposure dose, the greater the _____ of cancer.

4. Many scientists in the early years of radiation research developed a dry, red skin condition called _____.

5. All cancers are characterized by uncontrolled _____ and _____ of abnormal cells.

6. _____ and _____ are the two primary types of carcinogens.

7. The activation of _____ and the loss of _____ genes are considered to be two of the primary contributors of cancer.

8. The _____, which are formed from normal _____, direct cells to function abnormally (usually to reproduce rapidly).

9. Radiation can activate a proto-oncogene to produce a malignant cell in three ways: _____ mutation, chromosomal reciprocal _____, and gene _____.

10. Most genetic mutations resulting from irradiation are caused by _____ mutations, which in turn usually occur as an indirect effect of the _____ of water.

11. Reciprocal translocations between different chromosomes are associated with _____ (similar/different) cancers.

12. Gene amplification occurs when there are extra _____ of the _____ in a cell.

13. Name four common causes of the loss of suppressor genes: _____, _____, _____, and _____.

14. To properly assess the risk of radiation exposure, researchers must use data from populations that have received doses of ionizing radiation _____ than normal.

15. Studies of cancer incidence from Hiroshima and Nagasaki show that cancer risk is related to _____ at the time of exposure.

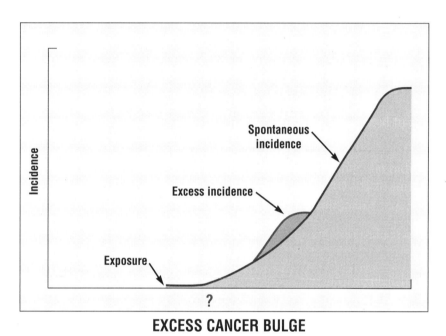

EXCESS CANCER BULGE

16. Absolute risk assumes a _____ dose-response relationship.

17. Researchers generally place cancers into two major groupings, based on where the cancer originates: _____ and _____.

18. Carcinomas represent _____% of cancer cases.

Module 5: Somatic Effects   101

19. Leukemia has a _____, nonthreshold dose-response relationship.

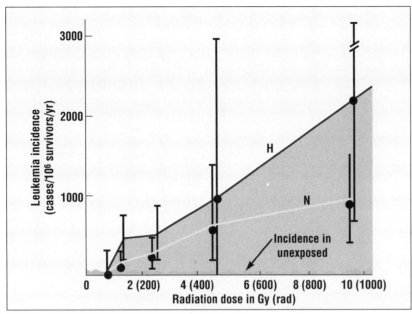

LEUKEMIA DOSE-RESPONSE RELATIONSHIP

20. Latent periods vary, depending on the _____.

21. Although _____ is the leading cause of lung cancer, a clear link exists between elevated doses of _____ and this deadly cancer. One of the greatest risks of lung cancer to nonsmokers comes from _____ gas.

22. Any dose of _____ is expected to _____ the risk of cancer.

Excess Cancer Mortality: Lifetime Risk/100,000, 0.1 Sv		
BEIR V cancer risk estimate for US population		
	Males	Females
Breast		70
Respiratory	190	150
Digestive system	170	290
Other solid	300	220
Leukemia	110	80
Total	770	810

Learning Quiz

Some of the following learning questions are similar to the interactive exercises found in the CD-ROM version of this module operated in the "Student Mode." Please provide the best possible short answer. The answers are at the end of this module.

1. Why is exposure to carcinogens only part of the development of cancer, not the sole cause?

2. Describe the process of cancer development.

Applications

The following questions ask you to apply the knowledge you have gained from this module. Please provide the best possible answer. The answers are at the end of this module.

1. Explain how studies of radiation-induced cancers differ from studies of radiation-induced hereditary genetic mutations.

2. Why did pioneering radiation researchers unknowingly increase their risk of developing cancer?

3. Explain the process of leukemia. Why is the name appropriate?

Posttest

Circle the best answer for each of the following questions. Your instructor has the correct answers.

1. What is the effect of radiation dose level on carcinogenesis?
    a. The higher the radiation dose, the more severe the cancer.
    b. Any dose increases the probability of cancer.
    c. The higher the radiation dose, the greater the probability of cancer.
    d. All of the above
    e. Answers (b) and (c) only

2. What is the radiation dose-response relationship of most cancers?
   a. Nonlinear, nonthreshold
   b. Nonlinear, threshold
   c. Linear, nonthreshold
   d. Linear, threshold

3. What dose of ionizing radiation does *not* increase the probability of developing cancer?
   a. 0.1 gray (10 rad) or less
   b. 1 gray (100 rad) or less
   c. 10 gray (1000 rad) or less
   d. 0

4. What is believed to have caused the death of Marie Curie, a pioneering radiation researcher?
   a. Old age
   b. Tuberculosis from patient exposure
   c. Leukemia from radiation exposure
   d. Chronic x-ray dermatitis from radiation exposure

5. Approximately what percentage of cancers can be traced to occupational exposure to chemicals or environmental pollution?
   a. 50%
   b. 80%
   c. 20%
   d. 5%

6. How much does smoking increase the probability of dying of cancer?
   a. No difference
   b. Twice as likely
   c. Three times as likely
   d. Ten times as likely

7. What is the normal activity of a cancer?
   a. Remains in one place in the body
   b. Spreads to other parts of the body through the bloodstream or lymphatic system
   c. Spreads only into adjacent organs through physical contact
   d. Answers (a) and (b) only
   e. Answers (a) and (c) only

8. Which of the following affects the *process* of developing cancer?
   a. Environmental versus chemical exposure
   b. Radiation dose
   c. Number of carcinogens contacted
   d. All of the above
   e. None of the above

9. How can radiation exposure activate oncogenes?
   a. Through gene amplification
   b. By chromosomal reciprocal translocation
   c. From a point mutation
   d. All of the above

10. Why is the normal expectation of cancer higher among men than women?
    a. More men smoke than women.
    b. Men face more occupational hazards than women.
    c. Women benefit from a natural protection that results from giving birth.
    d. All of the above
    e. Answers (a) and (b) only

11. Why is the risk of developing cancer greater if a person is exposed to ionizing radiation when young rather than when old?
    a. Natural defenses are weaker in youth.
    b. With older individuals, natural death may occur before the end of the latent period.
    c. Preventive practices are less effective for younger individuals.
    d. The young are still growing.

12. What is the risk of death from exposure for workers exposed to 0.001 Gy (100 mrad) of ionizing radiation?
    a. 1 in 100
    b. 1 in 1000
    c. 1 in 10,000
    d. 1 in 100,000
    e. 1 in 1,000,000

13. What groups do researchers study to determine the effect of radiation exposure?
    a. Employees of nuclear testing facilities
    b. Populations exposed to low levels of nuclear fallout
    c. Populations exposed to high natural background radiation
    d. All of the above
    e. None of the above

14. Which of the following is *not* one of the most common sites for cancer to develop?
    a. Bone
    b. Blood-forming tissue
    c. Lymphatic system
    d. Skin
    e. Uterus

15. How does the radiation dose-response relationship of leukemia differ from that of other cancers?
    a. Leukemia is more prevalent at lower radiation doses.
    b. The risk of leukemia levels off at a certain radiation dose level.
    c. Leukemia has a linear radiation dose-response relationship.
    d. Leukemia has a linear-quadratic radiation dose-response relationship.

16. Why are different cancers more prevalent in different geographical regions of the world?
    a. Diet
    b. Environment
    c. Heredity
    d. Exposure to carcinogens
    e. All of the above

17. What increases the risk of breast cancer for women?
    a. Age over 50
    b. Previous case of breast cancer
    c. Childlessness
    d. First child after age 30
    e. All of the above

18. What percentage of breast cancers are thought to be related to gene amplification?
    a. 20%
    b. 33%
    c. 45%
    d. 95%

19. What is the overall 5-year survival rate of persons with lung cancer?
    a. 2%
    b. 8%
    c. 13%
    d. 27%
    e. 63%

20. What is the relative risk of developing skin cancer from a dose of 5 to 20 Gy (500 to 2000 rad)?
    a. 2:1
    b. 4:1
    c. 10:1
    d. 20:1

Answer Key

Answers to Pretest

1. c

2. b

3. d

4. c

5. d

6. b

7. a

8. a

9. d

10. c

Answers to Review

1. Damage, mutation

2. Carcinogenesis or cancer, mutations

3. Probability

4. X-ray dermatitis

5. Growth, spread

6. Chemicals, radiation

7. Oncogenes, suppressor

8. Oncogenes, proto-oncogenes

9. Point, translocation, amplification

10. Point, radiolysis

11. Different

12. Copies, proto-oncogenes

13. Ionizing radiation, smoking, chemical agents, sunburns

14. Higher

15. Age

16. Linear

17. Sarcomas, carcinomas

18. 85

19. Linear-quadratic

20. Type of cancer

21. Smoking, radiation, radon

22. Radiation, increase

Answers to Learning Quiz

1. Scientists believe that cancer is the end result of a series of events occurring within a cell. Although it is an important event, exposure to carcinogens is not the only event that must take place for cancer to develop.

2. First, a normal cell undergoes some sort of mutation—spontaneous or induced by a virus, chemicals, or radiation. Then this cell replicates, passing on the mutation to the next generation of cells. As more and more cells replicate, the individual cells develop into a cancer, such as a tumor or leukemia.

Answers to Applications

1. To study radiation-induced cancers, scientists can use data from human studies and animal studies (such as those involving leukemias). To study hereditary genetic mutations, however, scientists must rely on large-scale animal studies.

2. Although early researchers became aware that radiation exposure caused x-ray dermatitis relatively quickly, they were not aware that radiation also caused malignancies with a long latency period.

3. With leukemia, the bone marrow produces an abnormally high number of immature white blood cells. These immature cells crowd out normal, infection-fighting white blood cells, which leaves the body more susceptible to infection. The term *leukemia* means "white blood."

Radiation Detection and Measurement

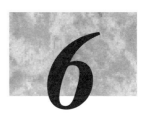

Self-Assessment Pretest

Before you begin to work through the Review, Learning Quiz, and Application exercises, use this pretest to assess your knowledge of the material in this module. Circle the best answer for each of the following questions. The answers are at the end of this module.

1. What is the traditional unit used for the measurement of radiation exposure?
    a. Curie
    b. Rad
    c. Roentgen
    d. SI
    e. None of the above

2. What is the primary source of radiation exposure for most people?
    a. Natural radiation
    b. Medical and dental diagnostics
    c. Radiotherapy
    d. Occupational exposure

3. How is the SI unit for exposure expressed?
    a. Watts
    b. Coulombs per gram
    c. Microcoulombs per kilogram
    d. Coulombs per kilogram
    e. None of the above

4. What is the basis for the National Council on Radiation Protection's exposure recommendations?
    a. Risk decreases as radiation dose increases.
    b. Threshold levels increase as radiation doses increase.
    c. No level of radiation exposure is safe.
    d. Each individual has a unique "safe" threshold level.

5. What is the purpose of personnel monitoring?
    a. To protect against exposure
    b. To provide a warning of excess radiation exposure
    c. To implement corrective measures
    d. To discipline employees

6. During routine radiographic procedures when a protective apron is not being worn, where should a personnel monitoring device be worn?
   a. On the back pocket below waist level
   b. On the front of the body at the waist or collar level
   c. On a wrist band
   d. A personnel monitoring device does not need to be worn.

7. What procedures produce a high risk of exposure for diagnostic imaging personnel?
   a. Fluoroscopy
   b. Special radiographic procedures
   c. Mobile radiography
   d. All of the above

8. What key action must be taken when a personnel monitoring device has been inadvertently exposed or lost?
   a. An estimate of true dose equivalent must be made.
   b. The employee should be disciplined.
   c. The employee should be enrolled in a radiation safety course.
   d. Answers (b) and (c) only

9. What are G-M detectors used for?
   a. To detect radioactive particles or photons in nuclear medicine facilities
   b. To determine radioactive contamination in an area
   c. To locate misplaced, lost, or hidden radioactive material
   d. All of the above
   e. None of the above

10. Which of the following is an area monitoring instrument used to measure the exposure rates (mr/hr) at various distances for a patient who has received a radioactive material for therapeutic reasons?
    a. TLD
    b. G-M detector
    c. Cutie pie
    d. Proportional counter

Key Terms

Before continuing, be sure you can define the following key terms.

Absorbed dose: The amount of energy per unit mass absorbed by the irradiated object; expressed in the SI unit—gray (Gy)—or in the traditional unit—rad.

ALARA: As low as reasonably achievable.

Centigray (cGy): One one-hundredth (1/100) of a gray; also equal to one rad. The centigray is replacing the rad for recording absorbed dose in therapeutic radiology.

Cutie pie: The nickname for an ionization chamber type of gas-filled radiation detector; one of the two primary types of gas-filled radiation detectors.

Densitometer: Instrument that measures the degree of blackening or density on radiographic film to determine the amount of radiation received and the energy of that radiation.

Deterministic effects: Biologic somatic effects of ionizing radiation that exhibit a threshold dose below which the effect does not normally occur and above which the severity of the biologic damage increases as the dose increases.

Dose equivalent (DE): The dose measurement that reflects the type and energy of an ionizing radiation, resulting in a measurement of the effective absorbed dose; expressed as sieverts in SI units or as rems in traditional units.

Effective atomic number: The atomic number calculated for human tissue, based on many various chemical elements of which the tissue is composed.

Effective dose: A measurement implying that the type of radiation and the variability of tissue and organs to absorb that radiation have been accounted for.

Exposure: The first key term in radiation measurement; expressed as coulombs per kilogram (C/kg) in SI units or as roentgens (R) in traditional units.

Exposure rate: The second key term in radiation measurement; calculated by dividing exposure by a unit of time.

Film badge: A personnel monitoring device that uses radiation dosimetry film held in a lightweight plastic film holder containing filters of aluminum or copper to measure whole-body radiation accumulated at a low rate over a long period of time (usually 1 month).

Gas-filled radiation detector: One of the two primary types of radiation survey instruments; uses a gas-filled chamber to measure radiation; capable of measuring the total quantity of electrical charge produced by the ionized gas or the rate at which the electrical charge is produced.

Geiger-Müller (G-M) detector: One of the two primary types of gas-filled radiation detectors; detects individual radioactive particles or photons; often used in nuclear medicine facilities.

Gray (Gy): SI unit for absorbed dose; named for Louis Harold Gray, a British radiobiologist; equal to 100 rads.

ICRP: International Commission on Radiological Protection.

ICRU: International Commission on Radiation Units and Measurement.

Linear energy transfer (LET): The amount of energy transferred on average by incident radiation to an object per unit of length of travel through the object.

Medical exposure: Radiation received during medical diagnosis or treatment.

NCRP: National Council on Radiation Protection and Measurement.

Occupational exposure: Radiation exposures occurring in the workplace and in the course of an individual's employment.

Personnel monitoring: Procedures used to estimate the amount of radiation received by individuals who work in a radiation environment.

Personnel monitoring report: A written report required by state and federal regulations to report occupational exposure; prepared by a monitoring company.

Pocket dosimeter: See *pocket ionization chamber*.

Pocket ionization chamber: A personnel monitoring device that uses electrodes to measure radiation exposure; also called *pocket dosimeter*.

Proportional counter: A type of gas-filled radiation survey instrument used in the laboratory setting to detect alpha and beta radiation.

Public exposure: Radiation from natural sources; includes all exposure not classified as either medical or occupational.

Quality factor (QF): A modifying factor for a given type of ionizing radiation that is used to adjust the absorbed dose value in determining the dose equivalent; also known as the *radiation weighting factor*. X-rays, which have a QF of 1, are the standard to which other types of ionizing radiation are compared.

Rad: Traditional unit for radiation absorbed dose; equal to 1 centigray.

Radiation survey equipment: A monitoring device used to indicate the presence or absence of radiation in an area.

Radiation weighting factor: See *quality factor*.

Rem: Rad-equivalent man; traditional unit for dose equivalent (rad multiplied by QF).

Roentgen (R): Traditional unit of measurement for exposure to x-ray and gamma radiation (named after Wilhelm Conrad Roentgen, who discovered x-rays in 1895); one roentgen is the photon exposure that produces—under standard conditions of pressure and temperature—a total positive or negative ion charge or 2.58×10^{-4} C/kg.

Sievert (Sv): The SI unit for dose equivalent; one sievert equals one joule of energy absorbed per kilogram of tissue.

SI units: Units standardized by the International System of Units.

Stochastic effects: Nonthreshold, randomly occurring biologic somatic changes in which the likelihood is proportional to the dose of ionizing radiation.

Surface integral exposure: Accounts for both the exposure and the area of the beam falling on the body of the individual who is being exposed.

TED: Total effective dose.

TEDE: Total effective dose equivalent; a radiation protection term that specifies the maximum allowable total accumulated dose.

Thermoluminescent dosimeter (TLD): Personnel monitoring device that uses a crystalline form of lithium fluoride as a sensing material to measure radiation; also known as *tissue-equivalent dosimeter*.

Tissue-equivalent dosimeter: See *thermoluminescent dosimeter*.

Tissue weighting factors: A value developed by the ICRP and adopted for use in the United States by the NCRP; assigns a relative risk factor for biologic responses associated with irradiation of different body tissues.

TLD badge: See *thermoluminescent dosimeter*.

Topical Outline

The following material is covered in this module.

I. Accurate radiation measurement is of utmost importance to anyone employed in the field of medical imaging.
   A. The International System of Units (SI) were adopted by the ICRU in 1980 for use with ionizing radiation.
   B. Radiologists and imaging professionals must be familiar with the standardized radiation quantities and units used today.
      1. Ionization of air is expressed in coulombs per kilogram (SI) or in roentgens (traditional).
      2. Amount of energy per unit mass absorbed is expressed as gray (SI) or rads (traditional).
      3. The dose equivalent for measuring biologic effects are expressed as sieverts (SI) or rems (traditional).
   C. Radiation exposure is classified in three general categories: occupational exposure, medical exposure, and public exposure.
   D. Variables in radiation measurement include exposure, exposure rate (time), and surface integral exposure (the size of the body area being exposed).
   E. The absorbed dose is the difference between the ionizing radiation entering the body and the ionizing radiation exiting the body.
      1. The absorbed dose causes biologic damage.
      2. The absorbed dose varies from one material or substance to another.
      3. The absorbed dose of a particular tissue or organ is calculated as the total energy delivered to an organ or tissue divided by its mass.
   F. Actual amount of biologic damage is related to the type and energy of the ionizing radiation.
      1. The effective absorbed doses of different types of ionizing radiation are indicated by the dose equivalent (DE) calculation.
      2. DE equals the absorbed dose multiplied by a quality factor (QF), a radiation weighting factor influenced by the linear energy transfer (LET).
   G. A measurement called the effective dose implies that the type of radiation and the variability of tissue and organs to absorb radiation has been taken into account through the use of appropriate weighing factors.
   H. Biologic effects of radiation are classified as stochastic and deterministic.

1. Stochastic effects are nonthreshold, randomly occurring biologic somatic changes in which the likelihood of the occurrence increases in proportion to the dose of ionizing radiation.
2. Deterministic effects exhibit a threshold dose above which the severity of the effects increases as the radiation dose increases.

I. The National Council on Radiation Protection and Measurements (NCRP) recommendations for limits on exposure to ionizing radiation are based on the assumption that no level of radiation exposure is safe.
1. The annual total effective dose equivalent (TEDE) limit has been set at 50 mSv (5 rem) for occupational exposure in any single year.
2. The NCRP recommends that a radiation worker's lifetime total effective dose (TED) in mSv should not exceed ten times that individual's age in years.
3. The NCRP recommendations are based on the principle of ALARA—"as low as reasonably achievable."

II. Knowledge about various personnel monitoring devices used to detect and measure radiation and exposure reporting is crucial to effective radiation protection.
   A. Personnel monitoring devices estimate the amount of radiation received by occupationally exposed individuals.
   B. Personnel monitoring is a warning, but it does not protect against radiation exposure.
   C. The primary methods of detection are ionization, photographic effect, luminescence, and scintillation.
   D. Personnel monitoring devices include film badges and ring badges, thermoluminescent dosimeters, and pocket ionization chambers.
   1. Film badges are the most economical and most widely used personnel monitoring device.
   2. Thermoluminescent dosimeter (TLD) badges are more sensitive—but also more costly—than film badges.
   3. Pocket ionization chambers, which provide an immediate reading, are the most sensitive of the personnel monitoring devices, but they are expensive and somewhat difficult to use.
   E. Personnel monitoring devices must be worn correctly to be effective, generally on the front of the body at collar or waist level. When a protective apron is worn, the monitor should be worn outside the apron at collar level.
   F. State and federal regulations require precise record keeping of radiation exposure in the form of a personnel monitoring report.
   1. Records of radiation exposure must accompany employees when they change jobs.
   2. Estimates of true dose equivalents must be calculated when monitoring devices are inadvertently exposed or lost.

III. Radiation survey instruments monitor areas to detect and measure radiation levels.
   1. Area monitoring devices measure the presence or absence of radiation. The detection system indicates the presence or absence of radiation, whereas the dosimeter system measures only cumulative radiation intensity.

2. Area monitoring devices can measure the total quantity of an electrical charge produced by the inonized gas and/or the rate at which the electrical charge is produced.
3. Most area monitors are ether gas-filled detectors or scintillation detectors.
    a. Gas-filled detectors generally used are either the "cutie pie" (ionization chamber-type survey meter) or the Geiger-Müller (G-M) detector.
    b. Scintillation detectors can detect a single photon interaction.

Review

Fill in the blank with the appropriate word or phrase. The answers are at the end of this module.

1. The principles of radiation protection are based on accurately quantifying _____.

2. The three primary guidelines for radiation protections are to minimize _____ time, to maximize _____ from the source of ionizing radiation, and to maximize the use of _____ materials.

3. Name the three radiation exposure classifications: _____ exposure, _____ exposure, and _____ exposure.

4. The greatest source of public exposure is _____ radiation. The greatest source of natural radiation is _____.

5. In simple terms, radiation exposure refers to the amount of _____ that may strike an _____. In radiographic terms, radiation exposure is the _____ of ionizing radiation delivered to a specific _____ of a patient's body.

6. Radiation measurement is based on the number of ion _____ in a known volume of _____.

7. The key variables in radiation measurement are _____, length of _____, and _____ of the patient's body.

Module 6: Radiation Detection and Measurement 117

8. As x-ray beam size _____, the amount of total exposure _____. The objective of radiographers should be to limit the size of the _____ to the smallest _____ possible.

9. Gy stands for _____, which equals one _____ of energy absorption per _____ of the irradiated material.

10. Rad stands for radiation _____ dose.

11. Radiation absorption is based on the _____ number of a material, its _____ density, and the _____ of the incident photon.

12. The extent of biologic damage is related to the _____ and _____ of the ionizing radiation.

13. Equal absorbed doses of different types of ionizing radiation produce _____ amounts of biologic damage.

14. The quality factor of x-rays = _____.

15. The dose _____ reflects the quality of different types of ionizing radiation.

16. One roentgen is equal to _._____ coulombs/kilogram.

17. The dose equivalent in rem is equal to rad multiplied by the _____ factor.

Radiation type	Absorbed dose ×	?	=	Dose equivalent
X-radiation	100 rad	× 1	=	100 rem
Fast neutron	100 rad	× 20	=	2000 rem
X-radiation	1 gray (Gy)	× 1	=	1 sievert (Sv)
Fast neutron	1 gray (Gy)	× 20	=	20 sievert (Sv)

118 Module 6: Radiation Detection and Measurement

18. According to the NCRP, annual TEDE should be limited to _____ mSv, but radiography students should not exceed an EDE of _____ mSv annually. Lifetime TED in mSv should not exceed _____ times an occupationally exposed individual's _____.

19. _____ and ring badges, _____ dosimeters, and pocket _____ chambers are the most commonly used personnel monitoring devices.

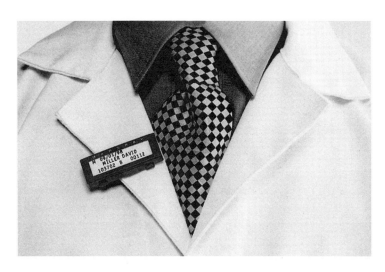

20. _____, _____ effect, _____, and _____ are the four primary methods of radiation detection.

21. Film badges can _____ if exposed to heat and humidity.

22. Thermoluminescent dosimeters are also known as _____ badges.

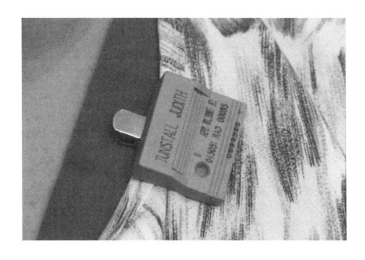

Module 6: Radiation Detection and Measurement   119

23. When two monitoring devices are worn during fluoroscopic or special procedures, one should be attached near the _____ and one is worn under the apron at _____. The badges must be _____ to avoid a mixup.

24. If an employee changes jobs, _____ records must be transferred to the new employer.

25. Area monitoring devices are known as radiation _____ instruments.

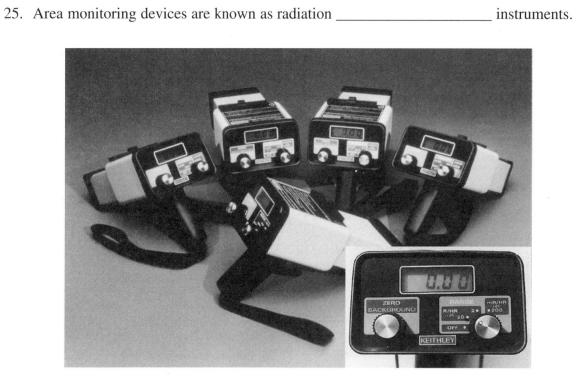

26. The two major types of survey instruments are _____-filled detectors and _____ detectors.

27. _____ counters generally are not used in diagnostic radiology.

28. _____ detectors are sensitive to radiation intensities as low as a single photon interaction, but they have a limited _____.

Learning Quiz

Some of the following learning questions are similar to the interactive exercises found in the CD-ROM version of this module operated in the "Student Mode." Please provide the best possible short answer. The answers are at the end of this module.

1. Explain how radiation dosimetry film is evaluated to learn about radiation exposure.

2. Describe the operation of a thermoluminescent dosimeter. Why is this device sometimes called a tissue-equivalent dosimeter?

3. Explain the operation of the pocket ionization chamber.

Applications

The following questions ask you to apply the knowledge you have gained from this module. Please provide the best possible answer. The answers are at the end of this module.

1. Explain the differences between stochastic and deterministic effects.

2. Describe the ALARA principle.

3. Summarize an effective personnel monitoring program.

4. Compare personnel monitoring devices to radiation survey instruments.

5. Explain the operating principle of scintillation detectors.

Posttest

Circle the best answer for each of the following questions. Your instructor has the correct answers.

1. Who discovered x-rays?
   a. Marie Curie
   b. Thomas Edison
   c. The International Commission on Radiation Units and Measurement
   d. Wilhelm Conrad Roentgen
   e. None of the above

2. When were SI units adopted by the ICRU for use with ionizing radiation?
   a. 1895
   b. 1985
   c. 1980
   d. 1904
   e. 1930

3. Which of the following is a source of radiation in the "public exposure" category?
   a. Workplace radiation
   b. Medical diagnostic radiation
   c. Radiation from natural sources
   d. Radiation from medical treatment
   e. All of the above

4. What is the greatest source of natural radiation?
   a. Radon
   b. Bricks and masonry material
   c. Cosmic radiation from space
   d. Tobacco smoke

5. What are the roentgen-to-coulombs conversion units?
   a. 1 roentgen = 3.88×10^3 coulombs/kilogram
   b. 1 roentgen = 2.58×10^{-4} coulombs/kilogram
   c. 1 roentgen = 2.58×10^4 coulombs/kilogram
   d. 1 roentgen = 3.88×10^{-3} coulombs/kilogram

6. What is the critical element in surface integral exposure?
   a. Patient health
   b. Patient age
   c. Radiation beam size
   d. None of the above

7. What is the absorbed dose?
   a. The amount of energy per unit mass absorbed by the irradiated object
   b. The total dose size
   c. The amount of energy of the radiation that enters the body
   d. The amount of energy of the radiation that exits the body

8. Which of the following *absorbs* the most radiation?
   a. Lead
   b. Bone
   c. Soft tissue
   d. Skin
   e. Organs

9. What is the dose equivalent value?
   a. Absorbed dose times SI unit
   b. Quality factor divided by SI unit
   c. Absorbed dose times the quality factor
   d. SI unit divided by the quality factor

10. What are stochastic effects?
    a. Randomly occurring biologic somatic changes with a specific lower threshold
    b. Nonthreshold, randomly occurring biologic somatic changes
    c. Nonrandom biologic effects with specific upper and lower thresholds
    d. Random biologic effects with a known upper threshold only

11. As determined by the NCRP, what is the average annual effective whole-body dose equivalent for exposed workers in the medical field?
    a. 15.0 mSv
    b. 15.0 Sv
    c. 1.5 mSv
    d. 1.5 mSv
    e. 0.15 mSv

12. What do film badge dosimeters measure?
    a. Radiation exposure to a specific part of the body from a single exposure event only
    b. Whole-body radiation accumulated at a low rate over a long period
    c. Whole-body radiation from a single exposure event only
    d. Whole-body radiation accumulated at a rapid rate over a short period of time, usually one week

13. If a film badge reveals excessive radiation from scatter, what could be the reason?
    a. Poor work habits
    b. Standing too close to a patient during a radiographic exposure
    c. A poorly designed radiographic facility
    d. Any of the above
    e. None of the above

14. What is (are) the advantage(s) of a film badge?
    a. Inexpensive, easy to handle
    b. Provides permanent record of personnel exposure
    c. Indicates direction from which the radiation reached the dosimetry film
    d. Simple to process without false readings
    e. All of the above

15. What is the sensing material used in thermoluminescent dosimeters?
    a. Radiation-dosimetry film
    b. Lithium fluoride in crystalline form
    c. Aluminum filters
    d. Copper filters
    e. Lightweight plastic

16. What is (are) the advantage(s) of a TLD?
    a. More sensitive and more accurate than film badge dosimeter; can be reused
    b. Measures a wide range of exposure and can be worn for up to three months
    c. Not affected by heat and humidity within normal ranges
    d. Answers (a) and (b) only
    e. All of the above

17. What is the measurement range of TLDs?
    a. 0–1.3 microcoulombs/kilogram
    b. 0–50 microcoulombs/kilogram
    c. 1.3–50 microcoulombs/kilogram
    d. 1.3–500 microcoulombs/kilogram

18. What is the sensitivity of pocket ionization chambers?
    a. 0–1.3×10^{-5} coulombs/kilogram
    b. 0–5.2×10^{-5} coulombs/kilogram
    c. 5.2–50×10^{-5} coulombs/kilogram
    d. 5.2–200×10^{-5} coulombs/kilogram

19. What is the primary advantage of pocket ionization chambers?
    a. Low cost
    b. Permanent dosage record
    c. Immediate exposure readout
    d. Resistance to temperature and humidity extremes
    e. Ease of use

20. What is the primary difference between radiation survey instruments and personnel dosimetry devices?
    a. Survey instruments cost less.
    b. Survey instruments provide instant readout.
    c. Survey instruments detect the presence or absence of radiation.
    d. Survey instruments can be used only once.

21. What is the "cutie pie" gas-filled radiation detector generally used for?
    a. To monitor diagnostic radiation facilities when exposure times of 2 seconds or more are used
    b. To measure the fluoroscopic scatter radiation exposure rate
    c. To measure exposure to patients who have ingested radioactive materials for therapy
    d. To measure cumulative exposure outside protective barriers
    e. All of the above

Answer Key

Answers to Pretest

1. c
2. a
3. d
4. c
5. b
6. b
7. d
8. a
9. d
10. c

Answers to Review

1. Exposure
2. Exposure, distance, shielding or protective
3. Occupational, medical, public
4. Natural, radon
5. Ionizing radiation, object or individual, concentration, area
6. Pairs, air
7. Exposure, time, area
8. Increases, increases, beam, area
9. Gray, joule, kilogram
10. Absorbed

11. Atomic, mass, energy

12. Type, energy

13. Different

14. 1

15. Equivalent

16. 2.58×10^{-4}

17. Quality

18. 50, 1, 10, age in years

19. Film, thermoluminescent, ionization

20. Ionization, photographic, luminescence, scintillation

21. Fog

22. TLD

23. Collar, waist level, coded

24. Exposure

25. Survey

26. Gas, scintillation

27. Proportional

28. Scintillation, range

Answers to Learning Quiz

1. The density or degree of blackening of the image recorded on the processed radiation dosimetry film is proportional to the amount of radiation received and the energy of the radiation. (A densitomer is used to measure this density.) To determine the amount of radiation the film was exposed to, the film is compared with the exposure value of a control film that was kept in a radiation-free area. The image can be evaluated to approximate the direction from which the radiation reached the film and to determine whether the radiation was caused by excessive amounts of scatter radiation. If high levels of scatter radiation are detected, the practices of the radiologist or radiographer and the design and procedures of the facility should be evaluated.

2. The thermoluminescent dosimeter, or TLD badge, generally uses lithium fluoride in crystalline form to measure radiation. When exposed to x-rays, the lithium fluoride molecules absorb energy, which is stored as excited electrons in the crystalline lattice. (The excited electrons are raised to a higher energy shell.) When the lithium fluoride is later heated, the excited electrons return to their natural orbit. As they fall back, they release energy as visible light. This light is proportional to the radiation energy absorbed by the TLD monitor. The atomic number of lithium fluoride (8.2), the material most often used in TLD devices, is close to the atomic number of soft tissue (7.4); thus TLDs are sometimes called *tissue-equivalent dosimeters*.

3. Pocket ionization chambers contain two electrodes, one positively charged and one negatively charged. When exposed to radiation, the air surrounding the positively charged electrode becomes ionized, discharging the mechanism in direct proportion to the amount of radiation received. Pocket ionization dosimeters must be charged before use. After use, readings are taken and the exposure should be recorded.

Answers to Applications

1. Stochastic effects are nonthreshold, randomly occurring biologic somatic changes in which the likelihood of the effect occurring increases in proportion to the dose of ionizing radiation. In contrast, deterministic effects exhibit a threshold dose below which the effect does not normally occur and above which the severity of the biologic damage (as opposed to the likelihood) increases as the dose increase. Cancer and heritable effects are stochastic effects; gastrointestinal syndrome, bone marrow syndrome, and cerebrovascular syndrome are early deterministic effects.

2. ALARA ("as low as reasonably achievable") is based on the belief that no exposure is safe. In following the ALARA principle, efforts should be made to ensure that radiation-producing equipment is well designed and used safely and that radiation exposure is properly monitored. The potential benefits of minimal exposure to ionizing radiation should far outweigh the potential risks.

3. In keeping with the ALARA concept, radiation workers who might receive about 1% of the annual TEDE (1% of 50 mSv) in a single month should be monitored. This includes employees of imaging departments, physicians, dentists, and anyone who performs portable radiography or portable fluoroscopic image intensification.

4. Whereas personnel monitoring indicates occupational exposure to radiation workers by detecting and measuring the quantity of ionizing radiation to which the dosimeter has been exposed over a period of time, radiation survey instruments monitor an area to detect the presence (or absence) of radiation. The purpose of survey instruments is not to report cumulative radiation exposure but to warn of elevated radiation levels.

5. Scintillation detectors contain crystals that emit light when they interact with x-radiation or charged particles. For instance, a single photon interaction produces a burst of light, which produces a photoelectric emission, which in turn is amplified to produce a large electron pulse. The size of the electron pulse is proportional to the energy absorbed by the crystal from the incident photon. Unlike TLD devices, which must be heated to release energy and produce light, the scintillation process occurs without heat.

Patient Protection

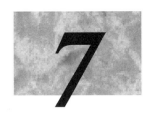

Self-Assessment Pretest

Before you begin to work through the Review, Learning Quiz, and Application exercises, use this pretest to assess your knowledge of the material in this module. Circle the best answer for each of the following questions. The answers are at the end of this module.

1. What is the first step to limiting a patient's exposure to ionizing radiation?
    a. Proper use of radiation protective shields
    b. Precise use of beam-limitation and filtration devices
    c. Effective patient communication
    d. Accurate exposure-factor calculations

2. What is the most common beam-limitation device in use today?
    a. Light-localizing variable-aperture rectangular collimator
    b. Aperture diaphragm
    c. Cone
    d. Extension cylinder

3. What should the primary goal of the radiographer be during a radiographic procedure?
    a. Reducing cost
    b. Making patient comfortable
    c. Minimizing patient exposure
    d. Limiting duration of procedure
    e. Ensuring patient convenience

4. Why are shadow shields used?
    a. For simplicity
    b. Because they are suitable for incapacitated patients
    c. Because they accommodate patients concerned with modesty
    d. Because they are appropriate when conditions must be sterile
    e. All of the above

5. Which of the following is true of intensifying screens?
    a. They reduce patient exposure.
    b. They reduce film exposure time.
    c. They convert x-ray energy into visible light.
    d. They enhance the action of x-rays on film.
    e. All of the above

6. What is the grid ratio of exposure factors comparable to using the air-gap technique?
   a. 1:8
   b. 1:80
   c. 80:1
   d. 8:1

7. Of the following, which procedure results in the highest patient dose *rates*?
   a. General fluoroscopy
   b. Orthopedic radiography
   c. Mobile radiography
   d. Mammography

8. What radiographic procedure results in the highest patient dose *rates*?
   a. Fluoroscopy
   b. Cinefluorography
   c. Mobile radiography
   d. Mammography

9. What is the simplest and most frequently used method of reporting patient skin dose?
   a. Entrance skin exposure
   b. Mean-marrow dose
   c. Genetically significant dose
   d. Glandular dose

10. What does the term *repeat radiographs* refer to?
    a. Any additional radiographs requested by a radiologist to obtain more diagnostic information
    b. A series of diagnostic or therapeutic exposures
    c. Examinations repeated because of human or mechanical error
    d. More than one examination in a 3-day period

Key Terms

Before continuing, be sure you can define the following key terms.

Added filtration: Filters added outside the glass window of the x-ray tube housing above the collimator shutters.

Air-gap technique: A scatter-reducing technique in which the image receptor is moved 10 to 15 cm away from the patient, which allows low-energy scattered x-rays from the patient to be absorbed in the air before reaching the film; an alternative to using a grid to reduce scatter.

Aperture diaphragm: A simple beam limitation device; consists of a flat piece of lead with a hole of a designated size and shape cut through it.

Beam-limitation device: Device that limits a patient's exposure to unnecessary x-rays by confining the primary beam to the area of clinical interest, thereby limiting the amount of body tissue irradiated.

C-arm fluoroscopy unit: Portable multiposition device used in the operating room for orthopedic procedures; produces real-time (motion) images of a patient.

Cinefluorography: Procedure using a movie-camera device (used most often in cardiology and neuroradiology); involves serial radiographic images that are recorded over a short period of time and then played back through a projector to allow study of motion within the patient (such as the spread of contrast media through vessels or the motion of structures within the heart).

Clear-lead shield: Shield (often used for breast and gonad shielding) made from a transparent plastic material impregnated with 30% lead by weight.

Cone: A type of beam-limitation device that confines the radiographic beam to a certain area; consists of a circular metal tube that attaches to the x-ray tube housing or variable rectangular collimator to limit the x-ray beam to a predetermined size and shape.

Elective booking: A method used to protect against irradiation of an unsuspected pregnancy; requires that the time of the patient's previous menstrual cycle be determined by the referring physician or radiologist.

Entrance skin exposure (ESE): The simplest and most frequently used method for reporting patient skin dose, usually measured with TLDs.

Extension cylinder: A type of beam-limitation device that confines the radiographic beam to a certain area; consists of a cylindric metal tube with a 10- to 20-inch metal extension at the far end of the barrel to limit the size of the useful beam.

Filtration: Elements that are part of, or added to, the x-ray tube to reduce exposure to the patient's skin and superficial tissues.

Flat contact shield: Uncontoured protective shield constructed of lead strips or lead-impregnated materials placed over a patient to protect areas of the body that do not need to be examined; available in a number of shapes.

Glandular dose: In mammography, the possible biologic response is related to glandular dose (which varies with variations in x-ray beam quality and quantity), not the skin dose.

Grid: Device that reduces scatter; made of parallel radiopaque lead strips alternated with low-attenuation strips of aluminum, plastic, or wood; placed between the patient and the film to remove scattered x-ray photons that emerge from the patient before they reach the film; improves image quality.

Genetically significant dose (GSD): The dose equivalent to the reproductive organs for the entire gene pool; if received by every human, this dose would be expected to cause gross genetic injury to the total population identical to the sum of the actual doses received by the exposed individual population members.

Inherent filtration: The glass envelope encasing the x-ray tube, the insulating oil surrounding the tube, and the glass window in the tube housing; amounts to approximately 0.5 mm aluminum equivalent.

Intensifying screen: Screen inside the x-ray film cassette that enhances the x-ray action by converting x-ray energy into visible light.

Involuntary motion: Motion that cannot be willfully controlled (e.g., when organs move or when an uncontrolled muscular movement occurs).

Light-localizing variable-aperture rectangular collimator: The most common beam-limitation device in use; contains multiple sets of lead shutters, one of which helps reduce off-focus or stem radiation.

Mean-marrow dose: The average radiation dose to the entire active bone marrow.

Mobile radiographic unit: Portable radiographic unit used when patients cannot be transported to an imaging department; requires a minimum source-skin distance of 12 in (30 cm).

Off-focus radiation: X-radiation produced by projectile electrons striking the anode at locations other than at the focal spot; also known as *stem radiation*.

Patient questionnaire: A method to protect against irradiation of an unsuspected pregnancy, in which the patient is asked to indicate her menstrual cycle.

Pigg-o-stat: A restraining device for infants used during radiographic procedures.

Positive beam limitation (PBL): Collimators with this feature automatically calculate the aperture (based on the distance from the film and the film size) so that the radiation field size matches the film size.

Phosphor layer: The active layer of an intensifying screen; the layer that converts x-ray energy into visible light.

Rare-earth intensifying screen: High-efficiency intensifying screen that uses elements with atomic numbers between 57 and 71 (such as gadolinium, lanthanum, and yttrium) in the phosphor layer.

Reflective layer: The layer of a calcium-tungstate screen that increases the efficiency of the intensifying screen by increasing the number of photons that reach the film.

Repeat radiographs: Any radiograph that must be performed more than once because of human or mechanical error in the process of producing the initial radiograph.

Source-to-diaphragm distance (SDD): The distance from the anode focal spot to the diaphragm opening.

Shadow shield: Shield made of radiopaque material suspended from above the radiographic beam-defining system; hangs over the area of clinical interest to cast a shadow in the primary beam over the patient's gonads.

Shaped contact shield: Protection device made of radiopaque material and contoured to enclose the male reproductive organs.

Shield: Device used to protect an area, such as the reproductive organs, from ionizing radiation; see also *clear-lead shield, flat contact shield, shadow shield,* and *shaped contact shield.*

Source-to-image distance (SID): The distance from the anode focal spot to the radiographic image.

Stem radiation: See *off-focus radiation*.

Thermoluminescent dosimeter (TLD): Device used to measure the entrance skin exposure for the purpose of assessing patient skin dose.

Voluntary motion: Motion controlled at will (e.g., skeletal muscle; when a patient moves all or part of his or her body, such as an arm or leg or the abdomen).

Wedge filter: Specialized filter that compensates for varying thickness densities of the foot; the thick portion of the wedge is positioned over the toes and the thin portion over the heel.

Topical Outline

The following material is covered in this module.

I. Effective patient communication is one of the most important techniques for limiting exposure to ionizing radiation.
   A. Radiographers should take a holistic approach to patient communications.
      1. Attempt to reduce anxiety.
      2. Educate the patient about the procedure, carefully explaining what the patient should expect to feel and hear, especially if the procedure will cause pain or discomfort.
      3. Elicit a patient's cooperation.
      4. Build trust between patient and radiographer.
   B. Poor communication can result in repeat radiographs and unnecessary exposure, often caused by patient movement.
   C. Be prepared before talking with a patient.
   D. Use clear, concise instructions and well-organized thoughts and routines.
      1. Use simple terminology that patients can understand.
      2. Take time to answer questions—and answer truthfully, in an appropriate tone of voice, in understandable terms, and within ethical guidelines.
      3. Listen attentively.
      4. Always consider the patient's age and ability to understand.
   E. Do not discuss concerns about a procedure with the patient, but do take concerns to a physician.
   F. Attempt to prevent movement.
      1. Voluntary motion results when a patient moves all or part of the body.
      2. Involuntary motion results when organs or muscles move.

G. Explain the need for, and methods of, restraint as well as the shielding devices to be used for the procedure.

II. X-ray beam-limitation and filtration devices limit patient exposure. Beam-limitation devices confine the primary beam to the area of clinical interest (thereby limiting patient exposure). Filtration removes low-energy x-ray photons from the beam, decreasing the intensity of radiation in the beam, which also decreases patient exposure.

A. Beam-limitation devices limit the amount of tissue irradiated (reducing patient dose) and help to improve image contrast.

B. Beam-limitation devices reduce the amount of scattered radiation.

C. Beam-limitation devices include aperture diaphragms, cones and extension cylinders, and collimators.

1. Aperture diaphragms control the size and shape of the x-ray beam. They are the simplest beam-limitation devices.

2. Cones of metal of varying lengths also control the size and shape of the x-ray beam. Now they are generally used for small field examinations of the head and sinuses and for specific views of the spine.

3. In addition to controlling the size and shape of the x-ray beam, light-localizing variable-aperture rectangular collimators also help reduce off-focus, or stem radiation.

D. Filtration decreases the intensity of radiation by absorbing some of the photons in the x-ray beam. Most of the lower-energy photons are removed from the heterogeneous beam, thereby reducing exposure to the patient's skin and superficial tissues.

1. Inherent filtration results from the glass envelope encasing the x-ray tube, the insulating oil surrounding the tube, and the glass window in the tube housing.

2. Added filtration, usually made of aluminum or its equivalent, is used outside the glass window of the x-ray tube housing above the collimator shutters.

3. The inherent and added filtration combine to equal the required amount of total filtration necessary to filter the useful beam adequately.

4. Compensating filters made of aluminum or lead-acrylic can be used to vary density of body tissue. These are inserted between the x-ray source and the patient to modify the quality or penetrating power of the beam across the field of view.

a. Wedge filters compensate for the varying density of body tissue.

b. Trough filters are used for chest examinations.

III. Shielding devices help minimize the body area exposed to radiation.

A. Protective shields should be used whenever a sensitive organ is in or near the x-ray beam.

1. Flat contact shields made of lead strips or lead-impregnated materials are placed over a patient to protect body areas that do not need to be examined.

2. Shaped contact shields made of radiopaque material are contoured to enclose body parts, such as the male reproductive organs.

3. Shadow shields made of radiopaque material cast a shadow over an area to be protected. These shields are suspended from above the radiographic beam-

defining system over the patient, and the beam-defining collimator light shows the position of the shadow over the area to be protected from the primary beam.

    B. Shields are made from a variety of materials, including lead, lead-impregnated materials, radiopaque material, and clear lead.

    C. The most commonly shielded radiosensitive areas of the body are the lens of the eye, the breasts, and the gonads.

    D. Shielding requirements sometimes differ between imaging facilities.

IV. Exposure factors, film-screen combinations, and grids are used to produce a useful radiographic image while minimizing patient exposure.

    A. Radiographers must balance patient exposure and image quality when choosing exposure factors.

    B. Film-screen combinations affect the amount of exposure a patient receives and the quality of the radiographic image.

    C. Grids are used to decrease scatter, thereby improving image quality but increasing patient dose. Even though patient dose increases with the use of the grid, the benefits obtained, such as improved radiographic contrast, makes the use of the grid a fair compromise.

V. Radiographers must apply special protection procedures for certain high-risk operations.

    A. The greatest patient radiation exposure rate occurs during fluoroscopic procedures.

        1. Protective shields should be used to reduce exposure whenever possible.

        2. Steps should be taken to limit the anatomical area exposed by properly collimating the x-ray beam to include only the area of clinical interest.

        3. The fluoroscopist should carefully monitor the length of exposure time the patient receives exposure using a cumulative timer.

        4. Patient dose should be carefully evaluated for each fluoroscopic procedure.

    B. The greatest patient doses occur during cinefluorography.

        1. Cinefluorography is most often used in cardiology and neuroradiology.

        2. Techniques used to reduce patient dose during fluoroscopy also apply to dose reduction during cinefluorography.

    C. Mobile radiographic units must be used selectively and with proper procedures.

    D. Mammography requires specialized equipment.

        1. Patient dose is important because of the radiosensitivity of breast tissue.

        2. Quality control—including testing, record keeping, maintaining and evaluating equipment, processing, and procedures—is extremely important in mammography.

VI. Understanding patient dose is a key aspect of limiting patient exposure.

    A. Imaging professionals must be capable of evaluating patient dose for various diagnostic procedures and balancing risk against the need for a given procedure.

        1. Entrance skin exposure (ESE) is the simplest and most frequently used method of reporting patient skin dose.

        2. Mean marrow dose is the average radiation dose to the entire active bone marrow.

B. Estimates of gonad dose (the genetically significant dose, GSD) are important because of the risk of genetic effects of ionizing radiation associated with gonadal exposure. The estimated GSD for the population of the United States is about 0.20 mSv (20 mrem).

C. The biologic response related to mammography is known as the glandular dose.

D. Radiographers should know how to protect higher-risk patients, such as children and pregnant patients.

1. Children require special protective procedures because they are more susceptible to both late somatic effects and genetic effects than adults.

    a. A useful image can be obtained with a lower dose of x-radiation for children than is needed for adults.

    b. Movement is more of a problem with children than with adults. Appropriate measure must be taken to eliminate, or at least minimize, motion.

2. Pregnant patients demand particularly attentive care because of the potential of exposing the embryo-fetus.

    a. The highest risk period for exposure to ionizing radiation is during the first trimester.

    b. Women often do not know they are pregnant during this high-risk period.

    c. Elective booking and patient questionnaires are used to help protect women who may not know they are pregnant.

E. Preventing repeat radiographs remains one of the most important goals for limiting patient dose.

Review

Fill in the blank with the appropriate word or phrase. The answers are at the end of this module.

1. A primary goal of every radiographer should be to _____ patient _____ to radiation.

2. Effective patient communication helps the patient be more _____, which can reduce the chance of the need for a _____ radiograph.

3. Effective patient communication works in two directions: Radiographers should not only _____ to patients, they must also _____.

4. Radiographers should never question the validity of an examination when talking with a _____.

5. Patient movement can be both _____ and _____.

6. Anyone who helps restrain a patient during a radiographic procedure must wear _____.

7. A restraining device used for infant chest radiography is called the _____.

8. _____ devices limit a patient's exposure to x-rays by confining the primary beam to the area of _____ interest.

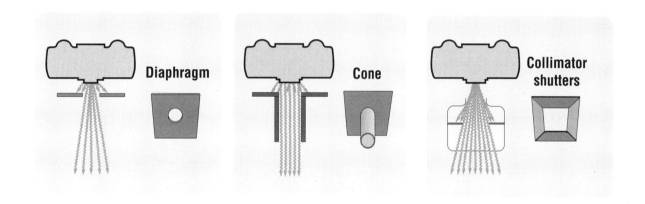

9. X-ray beams are restricted or limited to _____ patient dose and to improve image _____.

10. The diaphragm opening used depends on the _____ of the radiographic film and the _____ distance.

11. Beam limitation depends on the _____ of the tube and the _____ of the opening. Interference known as _____ results when the image is cut off as a result of mis alignment of a cone.

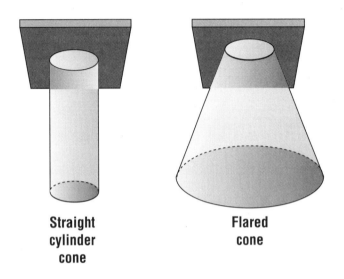

Straight cylinder cone

Flared cone

12. Positive beam-limitation (PBL) devices automatically determine what _____ should be used based on the _____ from the film and the film _____.

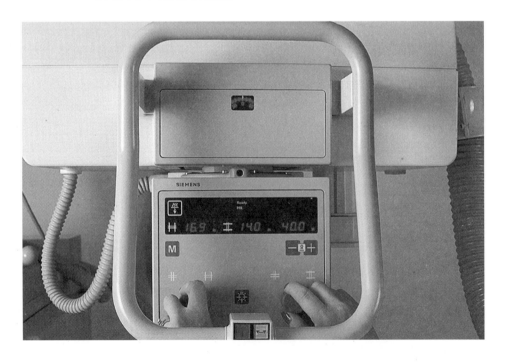

13. Because filtration increases the average energy of the x-ray beam, using a filter _____ contrast and _____ density in the image.

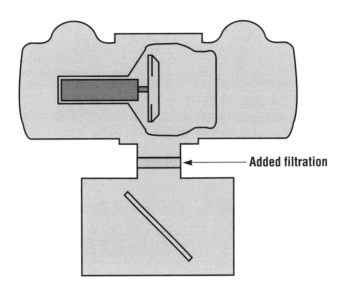

14. Protective shields should be used whenever a sensitive _____ is in or near the x-ray beam. The most frequently shielded areas are the _____, _____, and _____.

15. A flat contact shield used during fluoroscopy must be placed _____ the patient.

16. The correct exposure factor helps _____ patient dose while producing a _____ radiographic image.

17. Poor quality _____ = repeat _____ = unnecessary patient _____.

18. Patient exposure can be reduced by using _____ films and screens.

19. The use of the _____ can reduce scatter _____ (which can produce radiographic fog), which in turn helps the radiographer balance image _____ and patient _____.

20. The grid _____ indicates how effective a grid is at _____ scatter radiation.

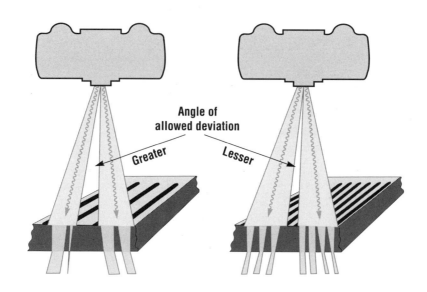

21. The _____ technique is an alternative to using a grid.

22. The greatest radiation exposure rate occurs during _____ procedures.

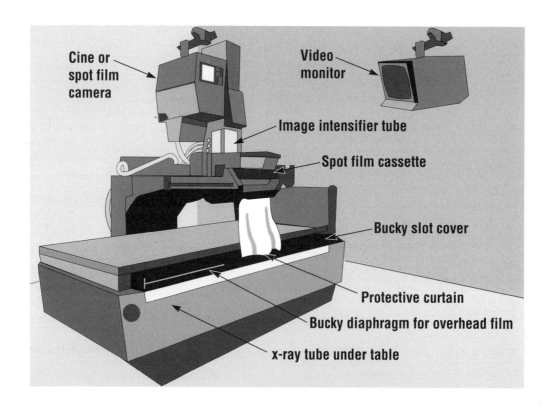

23. In mammography, as magnification increases, patient dose _____.

24. Assessing the _____ a patient will receive helps radiographers _____ exposure.

25. Active bone marrow in adults varies greatly from one _____ to another.

26. Measurements and estimates of gonad _____ are important because of the potential _____ effects of gonad exposure.

Estimated Genetically Significant Dose Caused by Diagnostic X-ray Exams

Population	GSD in mGy (mrad)
Denmark	0.22 (22)
Great Britain	0.12 (12)
Japan	0.27 (27)
New Zealand	0.12 (12)
Sweden	0.72 (72)
United States	0.20 (20)

27. The risk of an adverse biologic effect from mammography is considered to be _____ and _____ by the potential benefits.

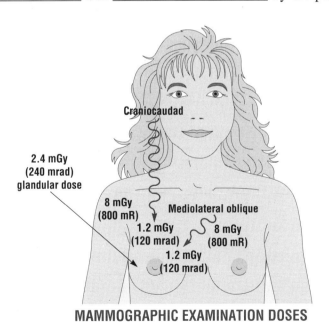

MAMMOGRAPHIC EXAMINATION DOSES

28. Two methods to protect against irradiation of an unsuspected pregnancy are _____ booking and use of the patient _____.

29. The concept of positive beam limitation (PBL) reflects a key principle of patient protection: The radiographic _____ should never be larger than the radiographic _____.

Learning Quiz

Some of the following learning questions are similar to the interactive exercises found in the CD-ROM version of this module operated in the "Student Mode." Please provide the best possible short answer. The answers are at the end of this module.

1. Describe how an aperture diaphragm functions. What is the correct beam area?

2. Explain how the relationship between the kVp, the mA, and exposure time is used to balance, producing a useful exposure with minimizing patient exposure. What tool is available to help radiographers balance exposure factors?

3. Relate grid ratio to the absorption of scatter radiation and to patient dose. What is the benefit of grids? What are the key selection criteria for grids?

4. Calculate the mean marrow dose if a patient received an average dose of 0.25 Gy (25 rad) to the bone marrow system and 50% of the active bone marrow were in the primary beam.

Applications

The following questions ask you to apply the knowledge you have gained from this module. Please provide the best possible answer. The answers are at the end of this module.

1. Describe effective patient communications.

2. Explain what a radiographer should do if he or she questions a procedure. When might this occur? What should a radiographer *never* do if a procedure is suspect?

3. Describe how the light-localizing variable-aperture rectangular collimator differs from aperture diaphragms, cones, and extension cylinders.

4. Explain how grids reduce scatter radiation. What effect does scatter radiation have on the image?

5. Discuss the different techniques used to limit radiation exposure during cinefluorography. In what situations does patient dose increase?

6. Explain how the compression device on mammogram units decreases patient dose.

7. Review the daily, weekly, monthly, and semiannual mammography quality control tasks that the radiographer is responsible for.

Posttest

Circle the best answer for each of the following questions. Your instructor has the correct answers.

1. What is the goal of an effective patient communication program?
   a. Alleviating the concerns of the patient
   b. Treating the whole person
   c. Educating the patient about the procedure
   d. Building trust between the radiographer and patient
   e. All of the above

2. What is a serious consequence of poor patient communication?
   a. Patient physical discomfort
   b. Inconvenience caused by scheduling misunderstandings
   c. Repeat radiographs
   d. Incorrect images taken

3. What steps should the radiographer take if the procedure will involve discomfort or pain?
   a. Tell the patient what to expect.
   b. Minimize the discomfort or pain greatly so that the patient is not frightened.
   c. Ask the patient if he or she would like to reschedule the procedure.
   d. Request that the referring physician be present during the procedure.

4. When should humans be used to restrain patients for radiographic procedures?
   a. Whenever possible
   b. Only for children
   c. Only when a mechanical support or device cannot be used or will not be effective
   d. Never

5. Who is responsible for limiting the x-ray beam during a radiographic procedure?
   a. The physician who requested the procedure
   b. The head of radiology
   c. The equipment manufacturer
   d. The radiographer

6. What is the simplest beam-limitation device?
   a. The aperture diaphragm
   b. The cone
   c. The extension cylinder
   d. The collimator

7. Why does the use of a cone improve the contrast of the radiographic image?
   a. The area exposed to x-rays is increased.
   b. Less detail is provided.
   c. Less scatter radiation is produced.
   d. The radiation dose is increased.

8. How does filtration reduce patient dose?
   a. By absorbing most of the lower-energy photons from the x-ray beam
   b. By decreasing the intensity of radiation
   c. By preventing low-energy x-ray photons from reaching the body
   d. All of the above

9. Why are specialized compensating filters used?
   a. To compensate for variations in x-ray beam strength
   b. To increase procedure speed
   c. To compensate for variations in the thickness or tissue composition of body parts
   d. To compensate for patient size

10. What is the common use of a trough filter?
    a. Neurological examinations
    b. Examinations of extremities
    c. Mammography
    d. Chest examinations

11. Which of the following is *not* a consideration in determining exposure factors?
    a. The effective atomic numbers and electron densities of the tissue involved
    b. The balance of radiographic density and contrast desired
    c. The type and quality of filtration employed
    d. The weight of any shielding devices

12. Where does the radiographer find the exposure factors for a given film?
    a. The radiographer must calculate the exposure factors using other known variables, such as SID and quality of filtration.
    b. The physician who ordered the procedure provides the exposure factors.
    c. The film manufacturer provides the proper exposure factors for each film.
    d. Generally, it is not necessary to be concerned with the exposure factors.

13. How does a grid affect patient dose?
    a. Dramatically reduces patient dose
    b. Can increase patient dose
    c. Has no effect on patient dose
    d. Affects patient dose only with repeat radiographs

14. How can patient exposure be limited during fluoroscopic procedures?
    a. Use protective shields to protect areas not of clinical interest.
    b. Properly collimate to limit the x-ray beam to include only the area of clinical interest.
    c. Ensure the proper exposure factors have been selected.
    d. Use a cumulative timer to monitor patient exposure.
    e. All of the above

15. What is the most common use for cinefluorography?
    a. Mammography
    b. Cardiology
    c. Setting broken bones
    d. Assessing scoliosis

16. What is the recommended minimum source-skin distance of mobile radiographic units?
    a. 1 foot
    b. 10 inches
    c. 1 yard
    d. 30 inches

17. Why is patient dose so critical in mammography?
    a. Patient discomfort
    b. Close proximity of the lungs
    c. The high radiosensitivity of breast tissue
    d. Patient anxiety

18. When using a dedicated mammographic unit for radiography of the breast, what is the benefit of magnification?
    a. Patient comfort
    b. Procedure speed
    c. Elimination of the grid
    d. Cost

19. Who is responsible for maintaining quality control in mammography?
    a. The radiographer
    b. The medical physicist
    c. The mammographer
    d. All of the above
    e. None of the above

20. In mammography, what level of repeat radiographs should trigger an investigation of the causes of the procedure failures?
    a. 20%
    b. 2 out of 100
    c. 5 out of 100
    d. 5%

21. How is entrance skin exposure usually measured?
    a. By calculating the exposure factors
    b. By evaluating the cumulative patient dose over a predetermined test period
    c. With a thermoluminescent dosimeter (TLD)
    d. All of the above

22. What is an important consideration in determining the genetically significant dose (GSD)?
    a. Type of examination
    b. Gonad dose per exam
    c. Age
    d. Gender
    e. All of the above

23. At what point is an embryo-fetus at greatest risk?
    a. During the first trimester
    b. During the second trimester
    c. During the third trimester
    d. At equal risk throughout pregnancy

Answer Key

Answers to Pretest

1. c

2. a

3. c

4. e

5. e

6. d

7. b

8. a

9. a

10. c

Answers to Review

1. Minimize, exposure
2. Cooperative, repeat
3. Talk, listen
4. Patient
5. Voluntary, involuntary
6. Protective garments
7. Pigg-o-stat
8. Beam-limitation, clinical
9. Reduce, contrast
10. Size, source-to-image
11. Length, diameter, cone cutting
12. Aperture, distance, size
13. Increases, decreases
14. Organ, lens of the eye, breasts, gonads
15. Under
16. Minimize, useful
17. Radiographs, radiographs, exposure
18. High-speed
19. Grid, radiation, quality, dose
20. Ratio, absorbing
21. Air-gap
22. Fluoroscopic
23. Increases

24. Dose, limit

25. Location

26. Dose, genetic

27. Small, outweighed

28. Elective, questionnaire

29. Beam, film

Answers to Learning Quiz

1. The size and shape of the hole determines the size and shape of the x-ray beam: the smaller the hole, the smaller the area exposed to the primary beam. The aperture diaphragm is placed directly below the window of the x-ray tube. The size of the aperture diaphragm is based on the size of the film. When correctly fitted, the area of the beam will be 1 cm smaller than the radiographic film.

2. Increasing kVp and decreasing mAs results in a high-energy x-ray beam, which reduces patient absorbed dose but produces a poor-quality image. On the other hand, decreasing kVp and increasing mAs results in a low-energy beam, which increases patient dose while improving image quality. Radiographers can use the technique chart for specific types of exams to balance exposure factors to produce a useful image while limiting patient exposure.

3. Grid ratios range from 5:1 to 16:1. As the ratio increases, the ability of a grid to absorb radiation increases, image quality increases, and patient dose increases. Generally, the improved image quality is considered worth the added risk to the patient. The key selection criteria for grids are the size and shape of the body part.

4. The average dose multiplied by the percentage of the active bone marrow in the primary beam equals the mean marrow dose: 0.25 Gy (25 rad) x 50% = 0.125 Gy (12.5 rad).

Answers to Applications

1. Radiographers should always be prepared and well organized. An effective communications program should include clear, concise instructions that fit the age and level of understanding of the patient. Patients should be told what to expect during a procedure in terms they can understand. Radiographers should always listen attentively to patients and take the time to answer questions. Answers to patient questions must be truthful, understandable, and within ethical guidelines.

2. A radiographer should always discuss any concerns about the validity of a procedure with the physician who requested the procedure or with another appropriate medical professional. Justifiable questions about a procedure might occur, for instance, if a patient has suffered an injury to one limb, but the procedure has been ordered for the opposing limb. Radiographers should never discuss concerns about a procedure with the patient.

3. The light-localizing variable-aperture rectangular collimator has multiple sets of lead shutters. The uppermost set, which is mounted closest to the tube window, helps reduce off-focus, or stem radiation. The second set, which is mounted below the level of the light source and mirror, confines further the radiographic beam to the area of clinical interest.

4. Grids eliminate many scattered x-rays before they reach the radiographic film. Scattered radiation, which travels at angles other than right angles to the film, can fog or darken the recorded image. This detracts from the viewer's ability to distinguish between the different structures being radiographed.

5. The most obvious method of limiting exposure during cinefluorography is to limit the time the beam is on, but this technique must be balanced against the requirements of the procedure. Another method is to increase the film speed. Reducing the viewing mode and increasing the frames per second will increase the patient exposure.

6. As breast tissue is compressed, the tissue is spread out and the breast becomes less attenuating, which allows for a decreased dose.

7. Daily tasks include darkroom cleanliness and checking that film processors are operating at preset specifications. Weekly tasks include screen cleaning and the cleaning of the viewboxes. Monthly tasks include making phantom images to check the film density, contrast, uniformity, and image quality (the images should be viewed by the same person, on the same viewbox, under the same conditions, using the same type of magnifier, and at the same time of day) and checking on the mammography unit. Quarterly tasks include analyzing repeat mammograms and determining whether processed films have higher-than-acceptable residual fixer. Semiannual tasks include darkroom fog analysis, film-screen contact tests on each cassette, and breast compression device checks.

Radiographer Protection

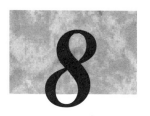

Self-Assessment Pretest

Before you begin to work through the Review, Learning Quiz, and Application exercises, use this pretest to assess your knowledge of the material in this module. Circle the best answer for each of the following questions. The answers are at the end of this module.

1. What is the whole-body annual total EDE limit, as set by the NCRP in 1993?
   a. 50 Sv (5000 rems)
   b. 5 Sv (500 rems)
   c. 5 mSv (500 mrems)
   d. 50 mSv (5000 mrems)

2. What is the primary source of scatter radiation during radiography and fluoroscopy?
   a. The protective housing of the x-ray tube
   b. The patient
   c. The radiographic film
   d. The primary protective barriers

3. Why is it best to place an x-ray machine in the center of the room?
   a. To optimize patient access
   b. To optimize radiographer access
   c. So all walls will be equally exposed to radiation
   d. To improve the view from the control booth
   e. Answers (a) and (b) only

4. What is the most effective means of radiation protection?
   a. Distance
   b. Shielding
   c. Barriers
   d. Radiation monitors
   e. Equipment timers

5. What is the occupancy factor for controlled areas?
   a. Always 1
   b. Depends on the use
   c. Zero
   d. Two or more

6. Where is the protective drape placed during fluoroscopy?
   a. Over the patient's pelvic region
   b. Over the fluoroscopist's shoulders and torso
   c. Between the patient and the fluoroscopist
   d. Under the patient
   e. On top of the patient

7. Where should the fluoroscopic exposure monitor be worn?
   a. At hip level, outside the lead apron
   b. Over the abdomen, outside the lead apron
   c. On the lab coat breast pocket under the lead apron
   d. Outside the lead apron at collar level
   e. At the waist, under the lead apron

8. What is the single most effective protective measure to take for someone acting as a human restraint?
   a. Keep the individual out of the primary beam.
   b. Have the individual wear protective garments.
   c. Have the individual wear protective glasses.
   d. Have the individual wear protective gloves.
   e. Make sure the individual has completed an occupational safety course on ionizing radiation.

9. What is the EDE for the embryo-fetus of a pregnant radiographer per month of gestation?
   a. 5 Sv (0.5 rem)/month
   b. 5 mSv (0.5 rem)/month
   c. 0.5 Sv (0.05 rem)/month
   d. 0.5 mSv (0.05 mrem)/month

10. What is the primary cause of x-radiation exposure to radiographers?
    a. Primary-beam radiation
    b. Scatter radiation
    c. Radiation leaking from the protective housing of the x-ray tube
    d. Radiation from the Bucky slot

Key Terms

Before continuing, be sure you can define the following key terms.

ALARA: The concept of radiation protection requiring that radiation exposure be kept "as low as reasonably achievable."

Beam-direction factor: Another name for *use factor*.

Bucky slot cover: A protective shield that covers the Bucky slot opening in the side of the x-ray table during a fluoroscopic examination when the Bucky tray is moved to the foot end of the table.

Clear-lead shield: Shield (often used for breast and gonad shielding) made from transparent plastic material impregnated with 30% lead by weight.

Controlled area: Areas occupied by employees who have been trained in radiation protection procedures and who wear radiation monitoring devices.

Cumulative timer: A radiation protection device used during fluoroscopy that either sounds an alarm or interrupts the x-ray beam after the fluoroscope has been activated for 5 minutes to ensure that the operator is aware of the "ON" time of the beam.

Declared pregnancy: A pregnancy that has been reported to a radiographer's supervisor.

Effective dose equivalent (EDE) limit: The upper boundary dose of ionizing radiation that will result in a negligible risk of bodily injury or genetic damage to the recipient.

Effective dose equivalent (EDE) limiting system: A system that provides a method for assessing radiation exposure and associated risk of biologic damage to radiation workers and the general public; this method determines the various risks of cancer and genetic effects to tissue and organs exposed to radiation.

Fluoroscopic exposure monitor: A monitor that emits a beeping signal directly proportional to the exposure rate—that is, the beeping speeds up and slows down as the exposure rate increases and decreases—to help the radiographer determine the best place to stand to reduce exposure.

Fluoroscopic exposure switch: A dead-man type of foot pedal that shuts off the x-ray beam if the operator becomes incapacitated during a fluoroscopic procedure.

General public: Patients, visitors, and anyone else not trained to work with radiation.

Inverse-square law: Law stating that the intensity of radiation is inversely proportional to the square of the distance from the radiation source.

NCRP: National Council of Radiation Protection; group that reviews regulations formulated by the International Commission on Radiological Protection (ICRP) and decides how to include them in U.S. radiation protection criteria.

Occupancy factor (T): A factor used to modify the shielding requirements for a particular barrier by accounting for the percentage of time that the space beyond the barrier is occupied.

Primary beam: X-ray photons that move in a straight-line path from the tube.

Primary protective barrier: Any wall to which the primary beam may be directed. It is designed to prevent primary radiation from reaching personnel or others on the other side of the barrier.

Primary radiation: Radiation from the useful beam.

Protective drape: A protective barrier used in fluoroscopy; consists of a sliding panel with a minimum of 0.25-mm lead equivalent attached to the front of the spot film device of a fluoroscopic x-ray unit for the purpose of intercepting scattered radiation before it reaches the operator.

Secondary protective barrier: Barriers designed to protect areas from secondary radiation.

Secondary radiation: Both leakage radiation from the x-ray tubing and scatter radiation.

Uncontrolled areas: Areas occupied by members of the general public.

Use factor: The proportional amount of time during which the x-ray beam is energized or directed toward a particular barrier; also called the *beam-direction factor*.

Workload: The radiation-output weighted time when an x-ray generator is actually delivering radiation; specified either in units of mA seconds per week or mA minutes per week.

Topical Outline

The following material is covered in this module.

I. To minimize exposure to ionizing radiation, radiographers must practice effective radiation protection procedures and use appropriate shielding to ensure adequate safety.

   A. Radiographers should follow the ALARA principle closely.

   B. Radiation exposure can be minimized by following the three cardinal principles of radiation protection. These principles focus on time, distance, and shielding.

   C. U.S. government standards for occupational radiation exposure follow NCRP recommendations.

      1. NCRP uses the effective dose equivalent (EDE) limiting system as a guide for both occupational exposure limits and exposure of the general public.

      2. EDE limits are established for whole-body exposure and individual organs.

   D. Effective use of protective shielding is one of the most important means of minimizing exposure.

      1. Shielding should protect radiographers from primary radiation—radiation from the useful beam.

      2. Shielding should protect radiographers from secondary radiation—leakage from the x-ray tube housing and scatter radiation.

   E. Protective structural shielding includes walls containing primary and secondary protective barriers. The x-ray tube must also have a protective housing.

      1. Protective barriers are designed either to protect from primary radiation (primary protective barriers) or from secondary radiation (secondary protective barriers).

      2. The x-ray tube must have a diagnostic type of protective tube housing.

   F. Radiation protection design considerations for diagnostic x-ray suites must include distance, occupancy, workload, and use.

      1. Distance can be used as the most effective means of radiation protection. The inverse square law can be used to reduce radiation exposure.

      2. Occupancy reflects the usage of exposed space.

         a. Uncontrolled areas are occupied by the general public.

         b. Controlled areas are used by personnel who are trained in radiation protection procedures and who wear radiation monitoring devices.

c. The occupancy factor is used to modify shielding requirements for a particular barrier.
3. Workload refers to the time an x-ray machine is actually delivering x-radiation. This quantity reflects the weekly radiation usage of a diagnostic x-ray unit.
4. For primary radiation, the use factor takes into consideration the amount of time an x-ray beam is energized or directed toward a particular barrier.

II. Extra precautions must be taken during fluoroscopic and mobile radiographic procedures.
   A. During fluoroscopic procedures, radiographers should use protective devices such as protective drapes or sliding panels, a Bucky-slot cover, a cumulative timer, a fluoroscopic exposure switch, and a fluoroscopic exposure monitor.
   B. During mobile radiographic examinations, radiographers should take special protective measures, such as wearing protective garments, using a 6-foot or longer cord leading to the exposure switch, standing at right angles to the x-ray scattering object (the patient) line, and using mobile protective barriers.

III. A number of protective devices are available for radiographers to reduce exposure to ionizing radiation.
   A. During some procedures, radiographers should don protective apparel, such as a lead apron.
   B. Anyone who restrains a patient during a procedure should wear a protective lead apron and gloves.
   C. Radiographers should use neck and thyroid shields during fluoroscopic and special radiographic procedures.
   D. Radiographers should consider wearing protective eyeglasses to help reduce scatter radiation to the lens of the eyes.

IV. Pregnant radiographers must follow special protective measures to ensure the safety of the embryo-fetus.
   A. When a radiographer becomes pregnant, specific safety procedures should be followed.
      1. The pregnant radiographer should immediately notify her supervisor to declare the pregnancy.
      2. The radiation safety officer should review the radiographer's radiation exposure history to determine what protective actions are necessary.
      3. The pregnant radiographer should receive radiation safety counseling.
      4. The pregnant radiographer should read and sign a form stating that she has received instruction and understands the safety procedures necessary to protect the embryo-fetus.
   B. A second personnel monitoring device can be worn at waist level beneath the protective apron to measure the exposure to the embryo-fetus. This equivalent dose limit should not exceed 5 mSv (500 mrem) for the entire pregnancy.

V. Many methods and devices for reducing patient exposure can also help reduce exposure to radiographers.
   A. Beam-limitation devices can reduce scatter radiation.
   B. An effective quality control program ensures that equipment is safe and operating properly.

Review

Fill in the blank with the appropriate word or phrase. The answers are at the end of this module.

1. The cardinal principles for minimizing radiation exposure focus on

   _____, _____, and _____.

2. The NCRP uses the effective _____ limiting system,

   abbreviated _____.

3. Any wall to which the _____ x-ray beam might be directed must have

   a _____ protective barrier.

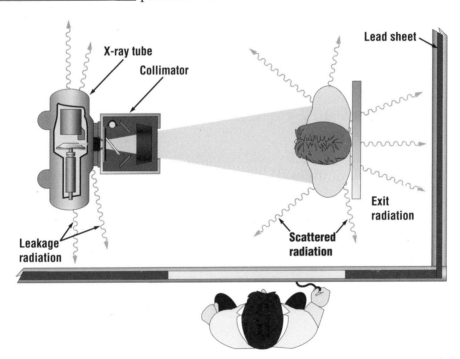

4. Radiographers should never point the _____ beam toward the control

   booth.

5. A primary protective barrier rarely needs to exceed _____ pounds per square foot

   of lead.

160   Module 8: Radiographer Protection

6. The high levels of radiation found in _____ medicine necessitate _____ protective barriers.

7. Secondary radiation includes _____ radiation from the x-ray tube and _____ radiation.

8. If the x-ray tube _____ has been properly designed and is not _____, leakage radiation measured at a distance of 1 m (3.3 ft) from the x-ray source should not exceed 100 mR/hr when the tube is operated continuously at its highest current for its full potential (voltage).

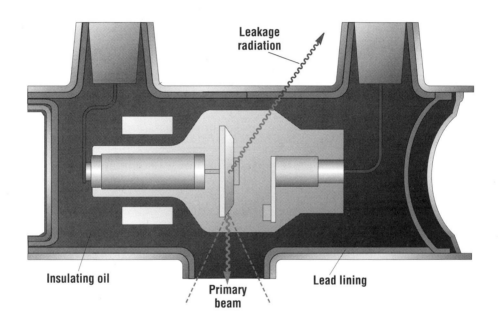

9. The glass viewing window of the control room generally is made of 1.5 mm of _____ glass.

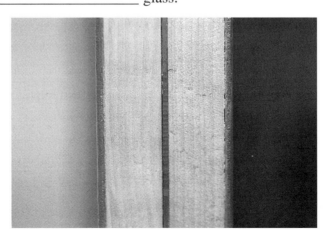

10. Doorways must be constructed as _____ protective barriers.

11. When designers calculate the required thickness of protective barriers, they must consider four factors: _____, _____, _____, and _____.

12. According to the inverse square law, radiation _____ is inversely proportional to the square of the _____ between the radiation source and the measuring point.

13. Occupancy in hospitals is considered to be either _____ or _____.

14. When the use of an area in a hospital changes, the _____ also changes.

15. X-ray rooms in which higher numbers of examinations are performed require more _____ than those performing fewer examinations.

16. When the Bucky tray is moved to the foot end of the table during fluoroscopic procedures, the resulting hole should be covered with a _____.

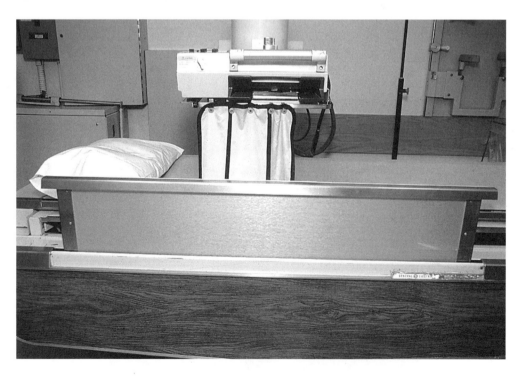

17. If the factors of shielding and distance are equal, the radiographer should stand at _____ to the x-ray beam and scattering object line.

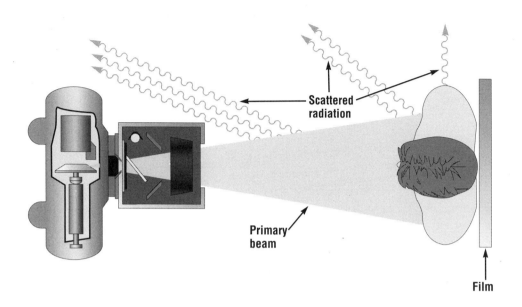

18. With mobile radiographic equipment, the exposure switch cord should be long enough to allow the radiographer to stand _____ feet away.

19. Radiographers should use _____ to increase their radiation protection during mobile radiographic procedures.

20. Rotating personnel is one method of reducing _____.

21. Protective gloves or mittens should have a minimum thickness of _____ mm of lead.

22. Wearing protective eyeglasses can help prevent exposing the _____ of the eyes to _____ radiation.

23. The equivalent dose limit for the embryo-fetus is _____ for the period of pregnancy.

24. A properly established quality control system monitors imaging _____ and _____.

Learning Quiz

Some of the following learning questions are similar to the interactive exercises found in the CD-ROM version of this module operated in the "Student Mode." Please provide the best possible short answer. The answers are at the end of this module.

1. Describe a properly designed control booth.

2. Explain the inverse-square law. If the intensity is 2 mR/hour at 3 feet, what would the intensity be at 6 feet?

Applications

The following questions ask you to apply the knowledge you have gained from this module. Please provide the best possible answer. The answers are at the end of this module.

1. Explain the cardinal principles of minimizing radiation exposure.

2. Review the precautions that a radiographer should take when she finds out she is pregnant. What are her exposure limits? What exposure monitors should she use?

3. Outline an effective quality control program. Who is responsible for the program?

Posttest

Circle the best answer for each of the following questions. Your instructor has the correct answers.

1. Practically speaking, what is the meaning of *ALARA*?
   a. Radiographers must avoid any exposure to ionizing radiation.
   b. Exposure limits are loose guidelines with a very high safety factor.
   c. Each person must decide what exposure limit he or she is comfortable with.
   d. Radiographers should strive to keep dose equivalent values below maximal allowable levels.
   e. Each facility with radiographic equipment must establish its own limits.

2. To what type of radiation exposure does the EDE system apply?
   a. Any and all radiation exposure
   b. Occupational exposure and exposure of the general public
   c. Occupational and patient exposure
   d. Patient exposure only
   e. Public exposure only

3. What are EDEs established for?
   a. Whole-body exposure
   b. Individual organ exposure
   c. Targeted skin-area exposure
   d. Answers (a) and (b) only
   e. Answers (b) and (c) only

4. What is the EDE limit during pregnancy?
   a. 0.5 mSv (50 mrem)
   b. 0.5 Sv (50 rem)
   c. 5 mSv (500 mrem)
   d. 5 Sv (500 rem)

5. Which of the following does *not* accurately reflect EDE dose limits?
   a. The limits are not above the approximate risk of death of persons working in "safe" industries.
   b. The limits are widely considered to be at an acceptable level.
   c. The limits represent the average exposure of personnel exposed to ionizing radiation.
   d. The limits are rarely exceeded by even one-tenth.
   e. The limits are rarely exceeded by imaging personnel.

6. In the design of protective structural shielding, what type of radiation is most hazardous and most difficult to protect against?
   a. Leakage from the x-ray tubing
   b. Scatter radiation
   c. Secondary radiation
   d. Primary radiation

7. Which statement below is *not* true?
   a. Lead shielding is specified in pounds per square foot.
   b. Shielding generally does not need to be greater than 4 pounds per square foot to be effective.
   c. 4 pounds per square foot equals a sheet of lead 1/16 inch thick.
   d. 12 inches of concrete = 1/16 inch of lead sheeting.

8. What is a common construction material for secondary barriers?
   a. 4 layers of 5/8-inch gypsum board
   b. Lead glass
   c. Lead acrylic
   d. 1/32-inch lead sheeting
   e. All of the above

9. What is the best location for the control panel exposure switch?
   a. On a very long cord outside the room where the radiographic equipment is located
   b. On a short cord directly outside the door to the room where the radiographic equipment is located
   c. On the wall next to the door inside the room where the radiographic equipment is located
   d. Either stationary on the control panel or on a short cord so that it can be used only from within the control panel

10. When considering the occupancy of rooms and areas, what does *general public* refer to?
    a. Patients
    b. Visitors
    c. Personnel who do not work with radiographic equipment
    d. Answers (a) and (b) only
    e. Answers (a), (b), and (c)

11. Why are secondary barriers always given a use factor of 1?
    a. They are constructed of less-protective material than primary barriers.
    b. The primary beam is not directed at them.
    c. Scatter radiation and leakage radiation are always present when the tube is energized.
    d. It is impossible to accurately calculate use, so 1 is used as a safety factor.

12. How can radiographers minimize their risk of radiation exposure during fluoroscopy?
    a. Place a protective drape between the operator and the side of the patient.
    b. Use a Bucky slot cover.
    c. Use a cumulative timer.
    d. Rotate personnel to distribute the exposure among several radiographers.
    e. All of the above

13. When using mobile radiographic equipment, where should the radiographer stand in relation to the patient and the primary beam?
    a. Directly opposite the center of the x-ray beam
    b. Directly opposite the front of the patient
    c. As close to the middle of the x-ray beam scattering object (the patient) line as possible
    d. At right angles to the x-ray beam scattering object (the patient) line

14. What protection devices should radiographers use during fluoroscopic and special radiographic procedures?
    a. A neck shield and thyroid shield
    b. A lead apron
    c. None of the above
    d. Answers (a) and (b) only

15. Who is the best choice for a human restraint during a radiographic examination?
    a. A radiographer
    b. Any person who has been trained in the radiation sciences
    c. An older relative or friend
    d. A young person within reproductive years who does not work with ionizing radiation
    e. Any hospital staff person who is pregnant

16. What is the EDE for occupants of controlled areas?
    a. 1 mSv (0.1 mR)/week
    b. 10 mSv (1 mR)/month
    c. Less than 1000 microsieverts (100 mR)/week
    d. 1000 Sv (100 R)/month

Answer Key

Answers to Pretest

1. d

2. b

3. c

4. a

5. a

6. c

7. d

8. a

9. d

10. b

Answers to Review

1. time, distance, shielding

2. dose equivalent, EDE

3. primary, primary

4. primary

5. 4

6. nuclear, primary

7. leakage, scatter

8. housing, damaged

9. lead-equivalent

10. secondary

11. distance, occupancy, workload, use

12. intensity, distance

13. controlled, uncontrolled

14. occupancy factor

15. shielding

16. Bucky slot cover

17. right angles

18. 6

19. protective barriers

20. exposure

21. 0.25

22. lens, scatter

23. 5 mSv

24. instruments, equipment

Answers to Learning Quiz

1. The control booth walls should be secondary protective barriers to intercept leakage and scattered radiation and should be positioned so that no one can enter the x-ray room without being seen by the radiographer. Also, the control panel exposure switch should be located so that it can be operated only when the radiographer is within the control booth.

2. According to the inverse-square law, the intensity of radiation is inversely proportional to the square of the distance from the radiation source. Thus, if the distance doubles, the intensity is reduced to one-fourth. If the intensity at 3 feet is 2 mR/hr, the intensity at 6 feet—double the distance—is reduced by a factor of 4.
   2 mR/hour ÷ 4 = 0.5 mR/hr.

Answers to Applications

1. The cardinal principles of minimizing radiation exposure focus on time, distance, and shielding. Specifically, the time of exposure should be kept as brief as possible, the distance between the source of radiation and the exposed patient should be as far as possible, and protective shielding should be used to block radiation.

2. A radiographer should immediately inform her supervisor to declare the pregnancy. The radiation safety officer should review her exposure history to determine what protective actions are necessary. She should receive radiation safety counseling. The pregnant radiographer should read and sign a form stating that she has received instructions and understands the safety procedures necessary to protect the embryo-fetus. As soon as the radiographer becomes pregnant, her EDE drops to 0.5 mSv (0.05 rem) per month. The equivalent dose limit for the embryo-fetus is 5 mSv (500 mrem) for the entire pregnancy. The radiographer should wear a personnel monitoring device at collar level outside a protective apron. A second monitoring device can be worn at waist level under the apron. This second monitor under the apron should show exposure values of less than 10% of those of the monitor outside the apron.

3. An effective quality control program will include acceptance testing of equipment when it is installed, routine performance evaluation, and correction of any problems. Performance evaluation should include filtration, collimation, focal-spot size, kilovoltage peak calibration, exposure timer accuracy, exposure linearity, and exposure reproducibility. Quality control should be a team effort, although the primary responsibility usually falls on the medical physicist.